HANGING
IN
THERE

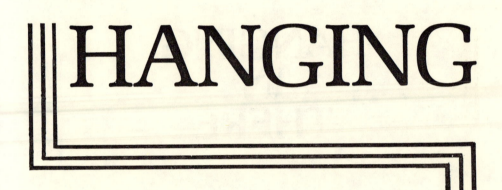

HANGING

IN THERE

Natalie Davis Spingarn

STEIN AND DAY/Publishers/New York

The poem "I reason, Earth is short " from *The Complete Poems of Emily Dickinson*, edited by Thomas H. Johnson, copyright © 1961, Little, Brown & Co., reprinted by permission of the publisher.

First published in 1982
Copyright © 1982 by Natalie Davis Spingarn
All rights reserved
Designed by Louis A. Ditizio
Printed in the United States of America
STEIN AND DAY/*Publishers*
Scarborough House
Briarcliff Manor, N.Y. 10510

Library of Congress Cataloging in Publication Data

Spingarn, Natalie Davis.
    Hanging in there.

    Bibliography: p.
    Includes index.
    1. Cancer.   I. Title.
RC263.S65   362.1'96994   81-48458
ISBN 0-8128-2866-6   AACR2

For my fellow hanging-in patients, past, present, and future: *Was mich nicht umbringt, macht mich stärker* ("That which does not kill me makes me stronger.")

—Nietzsche

CONTENTS

FOREWORD

For much of my adult life, I have written about health and social services for newspapers and magazines. After I fell ill with cancer in the early 1970s, I began to write in terms of my own experience.

I was struck by the response. You can write the most well-reasoned, well-documented third person story in the world, and people may or may not notice it. But write personally, about yourself, and the phone will ring off the hook for days, sometimes for months. It seems that though people hunger for health information, they respond most strongly to stories about individuals.

So I decided to expand what I had begun and try to address the relatively new problems of the patient who is, thanks to modern medical science, hanging in there with illnesses that once evoked only submission or surrender. Parts of what you will find in chapter 5 and to a lesser extent in the other early chapters have appeared in different form over the years since 1974 in *The Washington Post*'s "Outlook" section, and are reprinted by permission (the chapter 5 material appeared on September 13, 1981). But most of the material in this book derives from the burgeoning work on the psychosocial aspects of illness, and from my own, and other patients', experience.

I cannot begin adequately to thank all those who helped me in what we all hope will be a useful endeavor. Drs. Beatrix Hamburg and Stephen Hersh were good enough to read the entire manuscript, and offer me their suggestions; Dr. Hamburg has encouraged me from the beginning. Dr. Philip Cohen, social worker Grace Christ, and psychiatric nurse Lynn Brallier read parts of it. Gail Wilensky put her computers to work to glean new socio-economic information about cancer patients for me. Kathryn Kelly lent me her epidemiological, and Charlotte Crenson her health insurance, expertise. To them, and to the many experts and especially the patients who consented to be interviewed, my gratitude.

Thanks also are in order to my husband, Jerome Spingarn, who put up with me while I was writing, to Louise Des Marais, who so skillfully typed the manuscript while keeping an editorial eye out for the awkward phrase or misspelled word, and to Patricia Day, an expert and understanding editor.

Natalie Davis Spingarn

April 1982

CHAPTER 1

HANGING IN THERE

Living is what this book is about, not dying. Books about dying abound, some morbid, some inspiring, some useful—telling us how different people have died, or what phases we purportedly pass through as we die. Special shelves are now set aside for them in bookshops, as the poet-physician Lewis Thomas has observed, along with the health diet and home repair paperbacks and the sex manuals. Some of them tell personal tales of great fortitude; others advocate cures ranging from mind control to the (for me) counterproductive notion that you can conquer cancer by jogging or eating this way or that.

This book tries to take the matter a step further to address realistically the paramount issues for those of us who are, after all, still alive: living with serious illness, dealing with what that illness brings in matters both medical and nonmedical, without ending up as a burden to ourselves and those around us. It is neither a case history nor a medical tome. Rather, this book is the distillation of the experiences of the author, who is also a medical writer, and of others who have been through it all. It aims to be useful to patients and those who are trying to help them; to serve as a cheery gift one could intelligently present to a new, or seasoned patient.

3

"How are you?" people ask me, rather shakily and a bit curiously these days, knowing that I am being treated in a series of repeated bouts with cancer. "Hanging in there," I reply.

The statistics show that more and more of us are doing just that. In the early 1900s few cancer patients had any hope of long-term survival. In the 1930s, less than one in five were alive at least five years after treatment. In the 1940s, it was one in four. Now the ratio is one in three. The gain from one in four cancer patients surviving, to one in three represents about 70,000 people this year (1982), says the American Cancer Society (ACS).

More ACS statistics: Over 3 million Americans are alive today who have a history of cancer, 2 million of them with diagnoses five or more years old. Many of these 2 million can be considered cured. About 278,000 Americans, or about one-third of the people who get cancer this year, in the United States, will be alive five years after treatment.

The federal government's research center, the National Cancer Institute (NCI) adds that survival rates for seven of the ten most common forms of cancer have improved gradually since the early 1960s (cancer of the bladder, breast, cervix, large intestine, prostate, rectum, and the body of the uterus); not changed significantly were the rates for cancer of the lung, pancreas, and stomach. Memorial Sloan-Kettering Cancer Center, where I have enjoyed excellent treatment, is returning over half its patients to a "normal" life span. NCI director, Dr. Vincent DeVita, points out that cancer should no longer be considered "incurable"; in fact 45 percent of patients with serious cancers are alive five years after diagnosis, and by the mid-1980s the outlook for older (after fifty) patients should have improved as it already has for younger patients.

I have a healthy disrespect for statistics. I know from my experience as a bureaucrat in the higher levels of government, as a journalist, and as a sometimes public relations flack, that statistics can be used selectively to prove a point. I wonder, since I'm alive more than seven years after my first mastectomy, and since I've changed treatment sites several times, whether I'm showing up in some biostatistician's "cured" columns, though I've had recurrences. I know a great many of the new survivors are, happily, young people with blood-related diseases (Hodgkin's disease, for one).

Still, I believe what I see and hear, and I know there are many men and women now who, like me, are hanging in there. Some have had cancer and now suffer other diseases. My sister, for example, passed the five-year test after her mastectomy with flying colors, only to fall victim to rheumatoid arthritis. For years, she never thought about her mastectomy, she tells me. She thought a great deal about her arthritis, which forced two difficult operations to give her new plastic knuckles for her gnarled hands.

Of course, new drugs, surgery, and even new lifestyles have increased the life span of those who suffer from heart disease, stroke, and other killers. With our country spending about $1 billion a year in a war against cancer, and with my own experience, I have naturally focused on cancer patients. But I know patients who hang in with other illnesses.

A friend of mine who is a judge now goes about his job successfully after two open heart operations. Af first, the metal valve the doctors put in his heart smashed his blood cells so severely that he suffered spells of severe anemia. For a few years he elected to lead a quieter life, to cut his pace and take transfusions and medications when he needed them, rather than risk another operation. But repeated spells of terrible weakness changed his mind; he returned to the hospital so that the doctors could implant a new pig's valve in his heart. Now he is up and back on the bench again.

Sometimes those of us who are hanging in there do not have such logical, sequential choices, but I am convinced there are always choices one must make to survive. I had to make my first in the fall of 1974, when I opted to have a one-stage mastectomy instead of the newer two-stage procedure, but more of that

5

later. For two and a half years after that, I was home free—a little more bothered than the usual person about every little headache or belly cramp, but going about my business.

Then, in the spring of 1977, my upper back started to ache. I felt as though I had played tennis too hard and strained my back muscles. I waited for the pain to go away, but it didn't. I had a checkup; my internist said it was probably the familiar arthritis that had plagued my hip and knee, but, just the same, we'd do an x-ray when I returned from a press club trip to Europe. Between sightseeing forays in Portugal, I spent a lot of time chasing electric transformers that would enable my trusty heating pad to work on European current, and comfort my aching back. Back home in Washington, D.C., I faced the x-ray of my chest and spine, and another choice.

"You're not going to like this," my internist, Dr. Joseph Ney, warned over the phone as he described the radiologist's finding: In brief, something had attacked my upper spine, and I had suffered a collapsed vertebra. Several more consultations and scans confirmed that my cancer had evidently metastasized (traveled to another part of my body), specifically my thoracic spine (T-6). What to do?

The surgeon who had performed my mastectomy was retiring. I had to find a new doctor. Should I head straight for a radiologist or an "oncologist" (cancer doctor or chemotherapist)? Should I try for admission to the National Cancer Institute, the great research center in nearby Bethesda, which at that time, Joe Ney told me, was looking for breast cancer patients like me, with one metastasis?

Dr. Paul Carbone, then chairman of NCI's Breast Cancer Task Force Treatment Committee, had done a series of scans after my mastectomy and pronounced me fit. But my surgeon advised against going there. Referring to the Pennsylvania-based physician who was honchoing NCI's breast-research program, he warned, "You'll be taken care of by a computer in Pittsburgh." That was not quite accurate, but I understood what he meant. He wanted me to have more personal, flexible care than I would have had as a research subject, where my treatment would have been governed by a preset "protocol."

Some sort of wise genie stood up and whispered in my ear. I decided to go to a comprehensive cancer center for advice. There are 20 of these scattered about the country, and they are focal points, not only for research, but for the broadest and most skilled care and training available. I usually tell people who ask me how to get the best treatment to talk to their doctors about sending them to a comprehensive center nearby, if possible, at least for a consultation, be it Roswell Park Memorial in Buffalo, M.D. Anderson in Houston, or the University of Southern California in Los Angeles.*

For me, it was Memorial Sloan-Kettering Cancer Center, in New York City, where much of my family lives. I called Dr. Lewis Thomas, then head of that center, whom I had interviewed as a journalist. He said, "Come on up. I'd like you to see Dr. Thomas Fahey. He's an internist, and a good one. We'll start there."

I liked Tom Fahey right away. Not only was he a competent, humane internist, but a skilled endocrinologist and oncologist. He knew as much as there was to know about cancer, I could see that on my first visit. And he was not above drawing his own blood samples from my arm.

After going over me and my records thoroughly, he prescribed radiation to my back, "Let's sterilize that area first." After that was done (it was to take six or seven weeks), he strongly recommended an oöphorectomy, which meant he wanted to take out my ovaries and give me an instant menopause (I was past fifty and still menstruating, with little sign of stopping). I agreed to both.

I was to have the radiotherapy in Washington, D.C., with Tom Fahey continuing to supervise my treatment. Satisfied, I returned home. Like most patients, I felt better knowing some-

*For a list, and for information about other specialized institutions recommended for your case, call the federal government's Cancer Information Service. 800-638-6694.

thing was to be done—even if it was formidable treatment—to enable me to hang in. For how long? I did not know. But I felt I had maintained a certain amount of control over my situation. I remembered a story one of the Washington doctors told me about a woman with a back metastasis similar to mine who was feeling better in Iceland seven years after her cancer was diagnosed. There was a certain upbeat swing to that tale. I liked it.

When I first saw large numbers of little bald-headed, scrawny children with cancer at Sloan-Kettering, I thought their hanging-in problems were pitiful, but different from mine. Because they had lived shorter lives, they had a different perspective. Their lot was unfair, too, but I felt that since they had made less investment in the future, they generally had fewer potential dividends to lose—like my yearning to live to see my grandchildren.

Perhaps, I thought, there is more of a similarity to the parents of those poignant little people, who could seem so unlovable just when they needed love most. After all, these hanging-in parents, like me, faced an uncertain future. They, like me, were in danger of losing one of their most important investments in life, some of their most cherished goals. But gradually I have come to feel that though the hanging-in children's problems are different from my own, there is a similarity with them too.

In *There Is a Rainbow Behind Every Dark Cloud*, a group of California children with cancer write about choices in helping themselves feel happy "inside," despite what's going on "outside." They say you can speak up and say what's on your mind; you can cry; you can be mad at the world, and you can be afraid of death. You can use your imagination to fight disease; for them, this meant accepting their situation and expressing their feelings about it in drawings and through dreams, as well as conversation. I too have chosen to make myself feel better "inside" by trying realistically to accept what has happened and by speaking and writing forthrightly about my disease.

Above all, this means acceptance of the fact that though life

8

does not stop or change just because I am hanging in there, it is different. I have found I am now part of a subculture measured, not on an economic chart or sociological grid, but on a health progress chart. According to this "Criteria for Performance Standards," which I first saw on the Oncology (cancer treatment) bulletin board at the George Washington University Medical Center, I measure somewhat less than 80 percent—*able to carry on normal activity with effort, but with symptoms of disease.*

This subculture of the not-well, not-beyond-the-pale, exists everywhere, and it is growing as new drugs and medical procedures stretch our lives. In the Capital, we live under special pressure to behave as others do, even to behave better. I had done well for another two years after my radiation treatment at George Washington University Hospital, and my Sloan-Kettering hormone treatment (the oöphorectomy and, a bit later, a new antiestrogen pill developed in England called Tamoxifen). Then, in the spring of 1979, my left hip started to bother me. I bore with the pain for some weeks, thinking my arthritis was acting up.

But the pain persisted and worsened. On a trip to Atlanta to see my mathematician son, Jon, who had begun to teach at Georgia Tech, I began to have trouble moving my leg in and out of cars. I flew up to New York, where Tom Fahey ordered a bone scan. Later that evening he told me the radiologist, and he, were upset. The tumor had evidently spread; the bone scan showed a "hot" spot on my hip. He wanted first to radiate my hip and then to start me on chemotherapy, "If we continue to chase this thing only with radiation, we won't be doing anyone a favor."

I stayed first in the hospital and then in "hospital housing" for the hip radiation, which was no big deal. I had to use a cane, but I was able to keep a date in May of 1979 to go to Chicago and receive the American Psychiatric Association's annual Robert T. Morse Writers Award, "for outstanding contributions to the public understanding of psychiatry."

It was a heady, and somewhat unreal, experience to leave the hospital and march in a wobbly way to a hotel platform to be

9

handed a bronze medal. (I had to give it back for a period because "psychiatry" was spelled wrong.) But it was fun. I got through the dinners and other convention trappings and made it back to Washington, via New York, to begin chemotherapy.

"In Washington," my bright, well-trained, young Washington, oncologist, Dr. Philip Cohen, told me, when he started my chemotherapy course that summer of 1979, "our patients are *busy*." His clinic makes an extra effort to keep us "busy" people from sitting around waiting for test results. We can go to the doctor on our way to work one day for blood counts and come back the next day for treatment. We can be helped to lead "a normal life."

"Normal-shmormal" wrote journalist Stewart Alsop in *Stay of Execution*, a bit dated medically now, but, still the best book I have read about a struggle with cancer. Try as hard as I can, I cannot go about my business like a "normal" person. I am still on chemotherapy. I still have aches and pains. Even when aches and pains are quiescent, I do not *feel* the way I used to feel. My energy level is not high. I have to be careful how much I do, and how I do it. I'm caught on the horns of a dilemma: If I work more than a few hours, take buses or the subway, drive, invite people for dinner, I can suffer a setback. If I give in to myself with too many long breakfasts in bed or naps after lunch, I can lose confidence in my ability to stay afloat.

Like the "Rainbow" kids, I have found that there are certain survival skills you learn as you go along, certain behavior you try to elicit from friends and relatives. The "Rainbow" kids stress dependence on others. So do I. For them this means dependence on other children, who, as they put it, talk the same language, and so could be more helpful to them than adults. I too have found it helpful to face the fact that though I am basically an independent person, I am now dependent on others. At times I need them to drive me or bring me supper. And I have often, but not always, found it helpful to talk to my hanging-in-there peers, to share their joys and sorrows.

The other side of the coin does not escape the California

10

children. They point out that when other kids tease you, you can either pay no attention, or fight them, or choose to see that they are really scared. I, too, have found that when my adult friends avoid or act strangely toward "cancerous" me, I can ignore them, or confront them with what they are doing, or choose to see that they are scared. At one cocktail party, after chemotherapy treatments began to make my hair fall out, I was talking to two women. One complimented me on my hairdo. I replied, "Oh thank you. It's a wig." The women disappeared into the canapés. I chose to understand that they were scared.

Just as important, too, the kids who saw there was a rainbow behind every cloud understand the necessity to, as one social worker I consulted put it, "Place yourself existentially"—try to figure out the meaning of living. They speak of the power of love and of prayer, of letting go of the past, forgiving everyone, not being afraid of the future, and knowing that this instant is the only time that counts.

I too find my illness forces me to view my life more critically and intensively, through the eye of a needle as it were, to sort out what I want to do from what I don't, and then to go ahead insofar as I can, and do it. There's one important difference. The children help themselves lose their fear primarily by placing everything in God's hands, while I help myself lose my fear primarily by keeping alive my hope in the future.

This is important because unlike most "normal" people we subculture members have to live with the persistent knowledge of our own mortality. "Background music" Stewart Alsop called that knowledge, and it is true that when I am occupied the fearful dark tones stay in the background. But they can blare forth, affecting my attitude and ability to get on with the business of living. Why bother to plan a trip if I may not be around to take it? or to look for work? or build an addition to the house? A bit differently: How can I bear to leave the beauty of that autumn tree? or the joy of good books and friends? Jealously: Why is she living into her nineties with her grandchildren and great-grandchildren around her? while I . . . ?

I have found no skill more important (no matter how it is gained) than the ability to believe in my survival, for at least a

11

bit longer. For this, I am dependent on how my fellow human beings—doctors and nurses, family and friends—talk to me and deal with me, and what they give me, be it comfort or new medical knowledge, even more than on some higher force. I need them to reinforce the hope that sustains my life.

Bethine Church wrote to me recently that I am quite right in feeling that the "cancer twilight zone . . . is a world that other people haven't lived in." Describing Senator Frank Church's fight with cancer thirty years ago, and their feeling that he then had only six months to live, she said that forever after he had been a different person. It had been somehow easier for him to do the things that needed to be done, and let the things that did not matter go. We are all different people during, and after, an experience with life-threatening illness.

The background music forces most of us toward a search for meaning. Some find strength in a deepened religious belief. In a time of trouble, they find a new relationship with God, or intensify an old one. It seems to me that such men and women who have found a strong, clear faith are the lucky ones. I spend a great deal of time trying to weave my thoughts together, trying to figure out what it's all about. But no one, certainly not I, could have put the difficulties of doing so as succinctly as that solitary poet, Emily Dickinson:

> I reason, Earth is short—
> And Anguish—absolute—
> And many hurt,
> But, what of that?
>
> I reason, we could die—
> The best Vitality
> Cannot excel Decay,
> But, what of that?
>
> I reason, that in Heaven—
> Somehow, it will be even—
> Some new Equation, given—
> But, what of that?

CHAPTER 2

THE BAD NEWS

The phone rings, "Is this Toots?" asks a distraught voice. I know it must be someone who knew me, but not very well, long ago. She pronounced my childhood nickname with a short *o* (as in "Tootsie Roll"), while my family and really old friends use the long *o* (as in loose).

I was right. A friend of an old friend was calling me because I was a supposed fountain of knowledge about breast cancer. She had previous biopsies and aspirations (wherein the surgeon withdraws liquid from a cyst); all had proven benign. Tomorrow she was to have a biopsy, but only a biopsy, of a particularly thick, threatening lump. Was she doing the right thing? Had she chosen her doctor correctly?

I helped her as much as I could. I did not know her physician and advised a consultation at a cancer center if the lump proved malignant. *(To conduct an effective transaction with the environment, says the coping literature, the patient must secure adequate information.)* I thought how much had happened since 1974, when I had my first operation. Then it was unusual to be offered the "two-stage" operation, wherein the surgeon does a diagnostic biopsy and studies permanent sections of the lump before he discusses therapeutic alternatives as to what to do next with the patient. Now it is the consensus of an authoritative National Institute of Health (NIH) panel that the two-step procedure should be done in most cases.

Some people delay in seeking a diagnosis. There is even a literature on this delay period, which in recent years has been called "lagtime." But there is no overall agreement on the kind of person who delays before consulting a physician or the chief psychological factor that makes her delay. Perhaps she just needs more time to get used to the threat of cancer, to mobilize her defenses. Perhaps, afraid of knowing the truth, she rationalizes it couldn't happen to her because there's no history of cancer in her family. She fears mutilation or death. She has a poor relationship with her doctor. She denies or represses painful information, for a cruel but practical reason: She's divorced and worries that without a breast she'd be less attractive to men, or she's thinking of changing jobs, and with definitely diagnosed cancer this might prove hazardous.

My friend, we'll call her Nora, was a delayer, at first. An extremely intelligent divorced woman, she seemed to me to be denying the symptoms of her disease. During the summer a doctor at a Cape Cod clinic assured her that a breast lump would probably prove to be benign, but she should check it out in the fall. She was buoyed by the clinic's failure to impart a sense of urgency. (Wrongfully it turned out; why cannot doctors and clinics be tactful, and not scary, but still forthright about what needs to be done?) Even in September, she delayed the check, saying so and so hadn't liked the doctor she intended to consult. At Thanksgiving dinner, another friend asked her how the lump had checked out; Nora admitted she had not yet gone to the doctor. "You *what?*" That shocked question got her to the surgeon in December.

Actually, a delay of weeks should not worry anyone. To be palpable (felt by the hand) a cancer has to have been developing in the breast a long time, perhaps two years. I was abroad when I felt a lump in the upper part of my right breast. I knew it was a new one since the doctor had checked my breasts a few weeks

14

before. I had been in Bucharest reporting the World Population Conference; now, in Jerusalem, my husband and I were exploring Israel. I remember how big and hard the lump felt, but Jerry, my husband, was reassuring, per usual. Admittedly the lump was there, but I had lumps before and they had proven benign. Why should this one be different? I took a tour of Hadassah Hospital and suggested to him, "They are so smart here; perhaps I should show them the lump?"

But he pointed out I did not want to be hospitalized in a strange country, away from friends and family. So we went on to Spain, where we visited old friends, Len and Betty Slater, in Menorca. As we walked through that quaint countryside, checkerboarded with stone walls and white cottages, I started to tell Betty about the damned lump I kept feeling in my breast; I knew she had had one explored in Barcelona, with good results. But I did not because I thought it might prove to be just another cyst, and I did not want to worry anyone needlessly.

Home again, I called my cancer specialist, Dr. Calvin Klopp, and was in his office that same September week. As my husband had pointed out in Israel, I had been going to this calm, cool surgeon for over a decade because I suffered from chronic fibrocystic disease (lumpy breasts); I felt comfortable with him and trusted him. I had been in the hospital several times for biopsies, and had numerous cysts aspirated in his office. If a lump came back after aspiration, he took it out (too much activity there); if it was hard, questionable, he removed it as a matter of course.

Somehow, Dr. Klopp seemed to know, and I seemed to know, that this time was different. He said I'd go into the hospital the next week and he gave me a choice, a choice I'd never had to make before. I could give him permission to proceed as he saw fit, do the biopsy; if the results were benign, fine, he would sew me up again; if they were not, he would go ahead and perform the sort of mastectomy he felt best for me (the one-stage procedure). Another choice, I could have the biopsy and let him close the wound and we could discuss the results. If he found a

15

malignancy, we would have a week or two to decide together what sort of treatment or operation I would have (the two-stage procedure).

This choice, which I now applaud, disturbed me in 1974. This was two weeks before Betty Ford, with her publicly acknowledged mastectomy, caused us to be engulfed in a tidal wave of information; it was before Happy Rockefeller's operations, before mass mastectomy consciousness raising, before most people knew there was any alternative to just placing yourself in your surgeon's hands and telling him to do what's best for you.

For a week I worried about the choice. I consulted my internist, who advised me against the two-stage procedure; he thought that the offer was a result of the increasing wave of malpractice suits against the profession. I talked to my sister who had had the operation; she credited women's-rights pressures for the new patient participation. I called my physician-brother, Nathan Davis, in Baltimore; he said you would have to go to medical school, perhaps complete residency training as a pathologist, to determine intelligently what treatment would be best for your particular cancer: You would have to know the meaning of the type of cancer you suffered, and its position in the breast.

I did not go to the library to do research on mastectomies, as some women do. But, wearing my reporter's hat, I did talk to a number of informed people and read what I could get my hands on: For instance, I read a pocket book *What Women Should Know about the Breast Cancer Controversy* by Dr. George Crile, a doctor who dared suggest that mastectomy might not be necessary in early breast cancer. And I watched as one who followed his advice, his wife, the writer Helga Sandburg, bared her lumpectomy scar for a nationwide television audience to show women they might fight cancer without losing a whole breast.

Nowadays, the number of alternatives the surgeon has to offer you as a patient has increased, as has the idea of patient choice making. The 1979 NIH panel recommended as current

16

treatment standard not the "Halsted radical" mastectomy that had been standard practice for some eighty years, but a total (simple) mastectomy that removes the breast, as well as the axillary lymph nodes under the arm, but preserves the chest muscles. My friend Diana Michaelis a few years ago elected another path: She had the lump removed from her breast, then traveled to Boston for six weeks of intensive radiation therapy. The trials of this sort of treatment are still going on; the NIH panel felt it still too early to judge their outcome. (In Diana's case, it did not prove too successful. The cancer recurred in her lung, and her radiated breast shrunk and shriveled.)

Back in 1974, I felt better, calmer, as I explored the alternatives Dr. Klopp had available to him. (Point number two from the coping literature: *Maintain emotional distress within tolerable limits and thereby maintain satisfactory physiological condition so as to process the information further and act on it.*) At the end of what seemed a very long week, I chose the one-stage operation. The surgeon removed my breast and dissected almost all my lymph nodes (this could be called a modified radical mastectomy). My choice was based largely on my faith in my doctor, since retired, who did, I estimated, between two and three operations a week (a total of almost 5,000 over a thirty-year career) and thus knew more than I about what would be best for me. And at that time I lacked the faith in my own ability to chose losing my breast.

Six and a half years later, I had the experience, and the ability, to chose the two-stage operation. I did not even consider the one-stage. Other things were different, too. Tissue could be, and was, removed by a needle from solid lumps, like fluid from a liquid-filled lump (not enough could be extracted in my case to make a pathological decision). There was more reliance on mammograms (x-rays of the breast) and sonograms (pictures taken by sound waves). I was not put to sleep for a biopsy; it was done under local anesthetic in the George Washington University Hospital In-and-Out unit. The staff acted as though they were removing an ingrown toenail.

The diagnosis was not completed until the pathological slides

17

had been sent to Sloan-Kettering for expert consultation, a matter of a few weeks. During all this time I was anxious. I was angry at a George Washington bureaucrat for not responding promptly to Sloan-Kettering's request for more slides. But I was in control, and we were proceeding step by step. I did not panic. (Point number three: *Maintain autonomy and freedom of movement—taking care to avoid the feeling that there is either one right way or no way out.*)

At least this sort of change in medical technology or procedure is subject to serious scientific trial and experimentation. Others, especially changes in medical attitudes, often are not. Ninety percent of the doctors responding to a questionnaire in 1961 said they preferred not to tell cancer patients their diagnoses. In the late 1970s the same questionnaire showed a complete reversal: 97 percent of those responding said it was their general policy to tell patients the truth. The team reporting this policy turn-about in the *Journal of the American Medical Association* (JAMA) deplored the fact that in 1977, as in 1961, "physicians were basing their policies on emotion-laden personal convictions," rather than on scientific studies of the effect on patients of what they say.

During breakfast at the American Psychiatric Association's annual meeting, I talked about the JAMA article with a psychiatrist, Dr. Edward Gottheil, who had led a Philadelphia medical team in doing just such a study. We agreed that what is said to the patient at the time a diagnosis is made is particularly important. It sets the stage, as it were, for how the patient and his family deal with the disease from then on. In fact, all the experts agree that preoperative counseling about the sort of therapies that are open to us is crucial.

I did not have any problem, I told him, either with the way my surgeon first told me matter-of-factly in the quiet privacy of his office that the hard lump in my breast needed exploring, or later when, still in his green surgical scrub suit, he sat down in my hospital room and reported he had removed my breast because the lump was malignant, "garden variety," small, but *there*.

18

He thought my chances were good because he had "gotten it all." (What he and other surgeons really mean, by "getting it all," according to Harvard Medical School psychiatrist and coping authority, Dr. Avery Weisman, is "as much out as possible, there may be more.")

While Dr. Klopp spoke, I listened numbly. The pain flooded my torn chest as I absorbed the news. When he left the room, I wept for my lost breast. But this surgeon, skilled at dealing with patients as well as at operating on them, had prepared me for my loss. What if he had not? What if he had conveyed hopelessness, instead of hope?

I think I would have been as despairing as many patients. I would have been ten times more vulnerable to such hopeless doctor-remarks as, "I've seen this go pretty fast," or (to another woman) "You won't die of this stomach cancer. But it's already spread here—see this x-ray?—to the liver." I would have been desolated instead of just appalled by the resident who bade me a postmastectomy farewell: I was sitting on a bench near a hospital nursing station, waiting to be dismissed, when he approached.

"How are you?"

"Okay." And then, because that didn't seem enough, "I get blue once in a while, but that's all. The doctors tell me a little postoperative weeping is par for the course."

"Ah," he answered. "You like to read, don't you?" he had observed the books and magazines on my bed.

"Yes."

"Well, you should read *On Death and Dying*."

Having consigned me to the grave, he allowed that the operation I had was often successful. Then he disallowed such optimism by going through Elisabeth Kübler-Ross' *On Death and Dying* thesis: At first, the dying person denies his situation, then feels angry, asking, "Why me?" Before he could develop it further through the bargaining, depression, and acceptance stages, my son grabbed my arm and steered me away.

My suspicion that modern doctor-patient communications need reexamination was confirmed by the study Dr. Gottheil told me about. I certainly do not favor keeping patients completely in the dark as to what disease they suffer; I am only worried about how much and how this information is conveyed. But Gottheil and his associates found that hospitalized cancer patients who were not aware of their diagnosis had no particular advantage over those who were aware of it. They were not more engaged or involved in life (measured, for example, by their expressions or posture or grooming), did not have more visitors, and indeed did not live longer.

This did not surprise Edward Gottheil because the word cancer is often equated with death, and the knowledge of impending death was once part of punishment meted out for criminal behavior. (Wasn't the novelist Dostoevsky emotionally scarred for life when he was marched into the prison courtyard and prepared to be "shot"?) And he has seen increasing numbers of psychiatric referrals among "informed patients." The knowledge of impending death, he has found, is attended by fear and depression as often as by courage and dignity.

The "sock it to 'em" recital of survival statistics and dolorous disease details seems to be peculiarly American. France's Dr. Lucien Israël, in his valuable book *Conquering Cancer*, reports that he remains skeptical of his American colleagues' need to tell their patients the "truth" straight out and leave them to digest the news; he has seen too many patients anguished by this practice. He feels French doctors—not so bugged by fears of being sued and the necessity of seeking "informed consent"—have, collectively, a more responsible position when they say, "You have a serious disease," instead of, "You have cancer."

A British physician at first thought the American tendency to share information with patients, even the details of blood counts, drug, and radiation doses "quite extraordinary, even wonderful." But, after a year, this British colleague changed his mind, reported Dr. Stephen P. Hersh, formerly with the National Institute of Mental Health and now codirector of a Medical Illness Counseling Center. He now feels drowning patients in information has become a "vehicle for *not* communicating, for *not* listening, for keeping them as human beings at a distance."

Another sort of drowning is inflicted on us patients by doctors who think out loud while they examine you. These physicians not only expose you to their full conclusions, they expose you to the full process by which they reach these conclusions. As your examination proceeds you hear all the malfunctions you might have, as well as those you do have, and you have twice as much to worry about. I lay recently on an x-ray room examining table for three hours, my bowels distended with barium, listening to a young doctor try to figure out why the barium was not getting beyond a certain point. When she finally reported the culprit had turned out to be a spasm, not a lesion, it was too late. I had already suffered the mental despair of a metastatic blockage (another operation and a colostomy bag).

How did it happen? Why are doctors so convinced of the necessity of taking us into their every confidence? Why do they employ such harsh, straight-from-the-shoulder rhetoric about diagnoses and prognoses? The threat of malpractice has something to do with the new all-out-truth trend, of course. So does our "macho" culture, with its emphasis on being able to "take it." (I have found that people react quite differently when asked if they themselves want to know the "whole" truth: "Sure would," as opposed to whether they would want their spouses or children to know: "Well, I don't know.")

University of Rochester psychologist Garry Morrow has pondered this issue. He ascribes the new total-truth trend to: 1) improved therapy, which gives the doctor more to offer the patient and so more to discuss; 2) increased dissemination of cancer news by the media which makes all the terms more familiar and provides the patients with hints as to what to ask ("Do you think it will go with me the way it did for Betty Ford? or Marvella Bayh?"); 3) the patient and consumer rights movements, which instill the desire to "know" in some patients; and 4) the development of cancer centers (it's hard to fudge about the word "cancer" when you've been referred to Memorial Sloan-Kettering Cancer Center).

Be that as it may, the Bible tells us that when a Syrian king sent a messenger to Elisha to ask whether he would survive his sickness, the prophet responded, "Go, say unto him, 'Thou shall surely recover'; howbeit the Lord hath shown me that he shall surely die." Hopefulness was to be maintained, not merely by withholding information, but by positive encouragement.

Human nature has not changed since Biblical times. Circumstances, improved alternative therapies, for example, may have changed and may make it necessary to explain complex choices to patients, so as not to withhold information. However, the importance of hope, that elusive sentiment, remains clear.

Hope, according to psychiatrist Dr. Avery Weisman, is a *learned* response, produced by optimism, expectation, recollection of past successes and failures, and augmented by supportive and successful examples. If hope can be learned, then it seems to me doctors must strive constantly and painstakingly to teach it. There is nothing we, their patients, need more.

The well-known psychosomaticist Dr. Arnold Hutschnecker underlines this fact. He holds that hope sustains life; conversely, hopelessness causes death. Hutschnecker reports many cases of the power of hope. Patients fight cancer, he explains, with hope—hope of a cure, hope of a chance to live longer. In his book *Hope,* he cites a study of two hundred patients, each of whom maintain at least a little hope, explaining that people without hope see no end to their suffering but those with hope have confidence in the desirability of survival. It's true, hope gives us hanging-in patients something to live for, it enables us to endure uncomfortable tests and tedious treatments.

Another expert, Johns Hopkins Professor Emeritus, Dr. Jerome Frank feels strongly that a patient's own recuperative powers can be enhanced by hope and faith. In civilized as well as primitive societies, he reports, a person's conviction that his predicament is hopeless may cause or hasten his disintegration and death. Why else is the death of aged people shortly after admission to state mental hospitals unduly high? What other reason than hopelessness, aggravated by abandonment, for the fact that no adequate cause of death is found at the time of their autopsy?

Writing in scientific papers, Dr. Frank tells about the striking results of a rehabilitation team who went into a chronic disease hospital that had previously warehoused "hopeless" patients with a program designed to change the atmosphere and give them hope that they could get better and get out into the community: Some 70 percent of the patients who had been hospitalized three to ten years left the hospital; 40 percent of them became self-supporting.

And psychiatrist Frank explains that the surgical operation, a single dramatic act that is expected to produce a prompt cure, has powerful psychological effects. An operation tying off an artery in the chest to relieve angina had good results; most of the patients experienced relief of their symptoms. But a mock operation in which only the skin was cut and the artery not cut produced the same results—disappearance of pain, enhancement of the quality of life, and improved heart function (as measured by the electrocardiogram).

Internist Eric Cassell relates that, when he was in residency training at Bellevue Hospital, in New York City, he had a midnight call from the psychiatric ward: An old woman was having difficulty breathing. He found the patient gasping for air, her skin blue from lack of oxygen; she had water in her lungs (full-blown pulmonary edema), resulting from a blood clot in her lung. He stood at the bedside feeling impotent, while a nurse went for urgently needed oxygen and drugs. The woman's face and her distress pleaded for help, so Cassell began to talk calmly but incessantly, telling her why she had the tightness in her chest, and explaining how the water would slowly recede from her lungs, after which her breathing would begin to ease bit by bit and she would gradually feel much better. To his utter amazement that is precisely what happened. Not only did her fear subside, but the noises in her chest disappeared under his stethoscope, giving objective evidence that the pulmonary edema was, in fact, subsiding. By the time the equipment came, things were already under control. The doctor had given the patient hope; they felt as though together they had licked the devil.

So without hope, there's no ball game. I repeat: I do not

23

contend that modern doctors and the medical teams they lead should keep every one of us patients in total ignorance of what is wrong with us and avoid discussing treatment with us. Far from it. Like my friend Dr. Gottheil, I think physicians should exercise caution and judgment in sharing information with seriously ill patients. They should be more careful in loading us with useless diagnostic, and even prediagnostic, information. They should tactfully and optimistically tailor their message and attitude to the individual—and we individuals range from the librarian, who feels more comfortable when she researches every single detail about breast cancer, to the Connecticut patient who, terrified by the minute description of a forthcoming coronary bypass operation, refused the operation, left the doctor's office, went home, and a short time later, died. (Neil L. Chayet, a Boston lawyer and Harvard Medical School faculty member, reported in 1976 that the doctor was then sued for "wrongfully causing" the death.) Until more research is done on how to communicate, doctors should arrange the facts like flowers in a bouquet, so they appear pleasing to the patient.

This is easier said than done. There are some tangible barriers that are, as is usually the case, most easily overcome. Several physicians have emphasized the importance of sitting down quietly with a patient, with no one else bustling around, for important discussions, as Dr. Klopp did with me but as Nora's doctor failed to do: He diagnosed her breast cancer and discussed alternative treatments smack in the middle of a busy hallway. Others stress the importance of the substance of the explanation itself. As Dr. Eric Cassell points out in *The Healer's Art*, "'You have a hiatus hernia' is a complete sentence in English, but not, if you will, in doctoring. To be complete for that purpose, the sentence must read, 'You have a hiatus hernia, which means that part of your stomach has been pushed up into the hole of the diaphragm through which the esophagus passes to join the stomach; and while this may cause you some discomfort, it is easy to take care of and will do you no harm.'" The doctor should tell what the trouble is, what it means in body

24

terms, and what it means in personal terms or what can be done about it.

Many experts point out that how information is conveyed is as important as what is said. On the West Coast, oncologist and internist Dr. Ernest Rosenbaum and his wife Isabella (who have written several useful cancer guidebooks) have found that patients are so anxious about a diagnosis of cancer that they have trouble concentrating on what is being said. At the doctor's office door, after a forty minute discussion of future tests and treatment, a patient was met by a cousin who asked, "What did the doctor say?" The answer: "I forgot."

Many studies have highlighted the frequency of the "I forgot" phenomenon. They show outpatients at a variety of treatment settings recall approximately one-half of what they are told.

This is why Dr. Rosenbaum offers new patients the chance to record the initial diagnostic interview. Then he gives them the cassette and loans them a player if they do not have one. That way, they can review medical explanations and instructions in a calmer, more rational moment. The doctor reports success with his audio-cassettes, which contain a "translation" in easy-to-understand language of the consultative letter he has written to the referring physician as well as a discussion of the nature and meaning of the disease.

Similarly, Rochester's psychologist Garry Morrow points out that doctors who want to communicate better with their cancer patients should be on the lookout for high anxiety, lengthy instruction, patient lack of knowledge, increased patient age, and lower patient intelligence—in that order.

Morrow's strategy for improving the readability of written documents includes the use of short declarative sentences, short words, and the avoidance of medical and legal terminology, or "Medispeak." Thus:

Grade A for: "I permit John Doe, M.D. and/or doctors and staff he may chose to do what is listed above. He can also use services like anesthesia, radiology, or pathology, if these services are for my benefit."

Grade C for: "I authorize and direct John Doe, M.D. and/or associates or assistants of his choice to perform the operation(s) or procedure(s) listed above including whatever incidental procedures and/or additional services, involving anesthesia, radiology, pathology and the like, as may be advisable for my well-being."

Particularly with oral medical information, Morrow suggests doctors give specific, definite advice, rather than abstract, obscure suggestions. He feels they should lead with the most important information; that they should categorize information, stress its importance, repeat it, and, again, use short words and statements. Instructions like "take this pill every evening after dinner" we remember better than "take this nightly." Plain words like "hair loss" and "heavy sweating" are remembered better than their medical equivalents.

The core of the matter is less technical. It is that we patients vary just as doctors do. We have different backgrounds, different tolerances for pain, different resources and family situations, as well as different attitudes and beliefs about this world, and for some, the next. Accordingly, even if we do not forget what the doctor told us generally, we tend to focus on certain key words, or "buzz" words, and blot out the rest.

My old friend and Vassar College contemporary Dr. Betty Hamburg, a skillful psychiatrist, now a professor at Harvard Medical School, is interested in "buzz" words such as "life expectancy," "guarded prognosis," "handicap," or "complications." She has told me it is hard to teach medical students how much information a patient can tolerate under stress. Confronted by confusing, contradictory medical predictions and choices, she explains, we patients have trouble absorbing abstract concepts no matter what our education or degree of sophistication. The likelihood of an information overload increases. In striking the difficult balance between informing patients as necessary, and burdening them with unnecessary, perhaps harmful, details, Betty Hamburg feels doctors have their biggest allies in us, their patients, if they will only listen to us.

For we invariably give clues as to what we want to know and how we want to know it. I said to Dr. Klopp at the time of my first mastectomy, "I'm paying you to worry about it; I don't want to worry about it" (meaning, "don't load me up with all sorts of statistics about my chances"). He caught on, "OK."

Another woman says, "My sister's doctor told her exactly what's up and she's off in the Caribbean" (meaning, "please tell me exactly what's what"). It's not even necessary to speak words to signal. We can just look away, avoid eye contact, or fall silent (Enough). We can head for the library (More).

Some physicians are simply more skilled than others at communicating. They understand more about "buzz" words, they are more sensitive to patients' individual sensibilities, and their need to maintain some sort of autonomy or self-control. Thomas Fahey, my favorite oncologist, explains carefully what's going on in my body and what we can and cannot do about it. He has a real talent for doing so in an unthreatening, morale-boosting way. He can say the worst things cheerfully, unfearfully. Thus I have a "crummy," not a "horrible," disease, or should my tumor "start to cook again," not "should it metastasize to the liver." And when I ask him something like, "How can you stand dealing with this awful disease every day?" he answers that "nice patients" like me help him do his job. That really makes you a managing partner in a difficult but controllable enterprise.

Lynn Brailler, the creative psychiatric nurse who runs the Stress Management Center in Washington, D.C., introduced me to what I call the "titering" principle. In medicine, to titrate means to put in a little of this, and then a little of that, until you achieve a comfortable balance. That is what I do with health information. I try to let the doctors know how much I want to know, and when. I usually can take just so much of the "sock it to 'em" statistics and predictions. I must balance them with hopeful information that highlights me, as a person, not a statistic.

Every case, after all, *is* different. "Miracles do happen," a very sick hospital roommate told me once, "maybe one will happen to me." I do not know if it did. But it could have, there are no rules. I'm told every experienced physician has seen an established cancer simply vanish. It's extremely rare, but it happens.

Why take away our hope that we may be among the lucky ones?

CHAPTER 3

BEING SICK: THE SHORT RUN

More years ago than I care to admit, when my son Jon was about to enter this world, I remember approaching the hospital reception desk and being asked all sorts of routine, inappropriate questions about who I was, what I did for a living, and why I was there. "I don't *do*, I *am*," one young mother-to-be I knew replied acidly in a similar situation.

Now a pleasant voice calls from the hospital a few days before admittance (even via long distance) to query you at length, gathering the necessary facts: name, rank, and serial number. Your hospital and health insurance is this voice's chief concern. Lord help you if you don't have any. But more about that in chapter 8.

The hospital! Once you would have entered thinking it was a place to die in. Once you would have shuddered at the thought of it, and all but abandoned hope when you were admitted. If you lived two hundred years ago, in Benjamin Franklin's time, his cornerstone inscription for the Pennsylvania Hospital was the best you could have said for it: "Piously Founded for the Relief of the Sick and Miserable. . . . May the God of Mercies Bless the Undertaking."

Today you are likely to consider the hospital a place to be born in and a place to be cured in, a haven during critical periods of your life. You go there dreading the worst, but in your heart of hearts, you expect the wonderful.

Medical progress has given you the chance to get not what you fear, but what you expect. It has also created a bewildering new high-tech world-unto-itself, which it pleases the social workers to call the "hospital ecology." In this high-tech world, as a part of the hospital ecology, you really start to hang in— even though you may have gotten the news of your illness earlier, in the doctor's office.

At the hospital gates you go through a battery of tests before you ever reach your room: chest x-ray, ECG, blood and urine tests. You can be passed from hand to hand efficiently and cheerfully and made to feel like a person, instead of a stiff body, by polite staff helped by a cordial volunteer (a former patient), as I was last time I arrived for an operation at Sloan-Kettering. Or you can be worried by a disorganized bunch of young para-professionals of varying quality. When I was being admitted for my first mastectomy in Washington, one young technician apologized for jabbing my vein repeatedly but fruitlessly after his lunch-time martini.

I used to smile weakly and tolerate such behavior. What was there to do but grin and bear it? But experience as a hanging-in patient has taught me there is indeed something I can do— nothing earthshaking, perhaps, but enough to help me, and the patient who comes after me, and the hospital itself. In brief, I can stand up for myself, act more assertively and responsibly.

This means I can say to the young man, not rudely, and not aggressively, but dispassionately and with respect for him and for myself, "I understand you're not feeling too great. How about finding a colleague to draw my blood?" Or "I really would feel more comfortable, and you might too, since you're having trouble today, if you found someone else to draw that blood."

This sort of asking politely, but firmly, for fair play helps when things do not go well in what for most of us is the enormous experience of hospital life. Generally we are unprepared for this experience. As middle-aged people, we may have been in the hospital briefly a few times over the years to have babies (happily) or to have our hemorrhoids repaired (a nuisance). We have not had to think hard, under the cloud of life-threatening illness, about today's hospital industry as big business, with its managers trying to operate it as such.

So you can be overwhelmed at the impersonality of hospital life. You can be dehumanized by the scene. Wherever you find yourself, whomever the staff, and whatever their training, your admission test results are correlated and computerized. In busy city hospitals, you are put to bed—filed, as it were—in a semi-private room, even if you ask for a single room and are willing to pay the noninsured difference.

Writing on his hospitalization in the prestigious *New England Journal of Medicine,* author Norman Cousins reported, "I had a fast growing conviction that a hospital is no place for the seriously ill." He must have been referring to the cool, sometimes seemingly mindless hospital routine: Waking you from a comfortable doze at 9:00 P.M., for instance, to take a sleeping pill. When he was a resident, a doctor I know went downstairs in a crowded hospital to take a much needed nap on the only available bed. Finding him there, an officious nurse insisted on waking him up and taking his temperature despite his protestations ("I'm a doctor! Not a patient!"). It was a good lesson for him.

For Norman Cousins, laughter is the chief answer, not only to the idiosyncracies of hospital routine, but to sickness itself. It is surely true that it helps to maintain your sense of humor, to gently kid your caretakers as well as yourself. This does not mean you do not take your serious situation seriously, just that you don't take yourself too seriously. In so doing, it helps to try to put yourself in the place of the bored housekeeper who runs her mop bumpily under your bed while she keeps her eye on your roommate's television "story," the aide weary from bedpan emptying or bed making who forgets to refill your water pitcher, or the nurse who takes the worldly belongings you need and locks them securely away.

31

With humor and empathy, you'll find it easier to speak up for yourself, tactfully "stroking" the other person before you state your suggestion: "That television story is absorbing I know, and a good diversion in the middle of your hectic day. But I'm feeling tired this morning, and I'd appreciate your turning it down while you clean the room." Or, "I know how busy you are doing a hard job, but I need some fresh water so I can take my medicines; I'd appreciate your getting it for me." Or, "I know you're locking my things away to prevent theft, but would you mind letting me keep my pocketbook for today because I need my eyeglasses and lipstick?"

Some patients fare well with hospital underlings, but become tongue tied when it comes to the higher ups. When your comfort, indeed your life, is in the hands of nurses and doctors, you are often afraid to assert yourself. You fear being thought pushy, or uncooperative. You feel the nurse and doctor may think you are ignorant or foolish, particularly if you "interfere" with their work or "take up their valuable time" suggesting changes or asking questions.

This is just the time you should speak up for yourself, asking the questions that are bothering you, and suggesting what seems sensible. The medical staff should know you are anxious. Doctor-researchers have told them many patients may feel fearful, even panicked, about cancer surgery, even though they know it ranks as the first and most effective treatment. Operating table mishaps are rare these days, but patients can dread them, worrying about what might happen under anesthesia. Dreams tell the story: One woman awaiting mastectomy surgery dreamt of seeing women's breasts hung on meat hooks in the butcher shop; another of women coming down the gangplank to have their breasts checked by a man at the foot; a man dreamt of seeing patients wheeled into a morgue.

Of course, not all of us patients experience the depression, anger, and resentment revealed by such presurgical dreams. But most of us feel somewhat nervous: We redo our wills and straighten our desks before we leave for the hospital. It is better for us and for our doctors if we share with them what's on our minds and ask for the information we need about our bodies and our lives, even if we just need to be reassured or to let off steam. Look at it this way: Your doctor may have been waiting for a cue from you as to what has been bothering you. You will be a "better" patient if you are better informed and thus more comfortable about what's happening. (But be sure your cue includes *how much* you want to know; you don't want to be drowned in a torrent of facts you don't need.)

My first mastectomy preoperation night was spent in a box-like hospital room next to the closet, with a blank curtain drawn between me and my roommate, who drew every agonized breath with difficulty. I spent a good many hours unhappily staring into the dark and silently stalking the hospital corridors. In contrast, last year when a group of residents kept me awake on a preoperative night examining my cantankerous roommate under bright lights, I spoke out, saying I understood how sick she was, but I would appreciate their trying to do their work more quietly and with fewer lights since I needed some sleep. They complied. I then asked for a single room and, the next day, got it.

Your chances for a cheerful, gallant outlook improve when you've adopted this approach. Another example: There is a good deal in the medical literature about treatment teams who work together to meet the patient's emotional needs and to avoid the fragmentation of care (a variety of doctors on a cancer team would include surgeon, radiologist, and chemotherapist; psychologist or psychiatrist, as well as nurse and social worker). But the reality is that the night before surgery you can be visited by as many as a half a dozen different caretakers who prod and poke and, vampirelike, draw more blood from you, ask repetitive questions, and insist that you sign "informed consent" forms agreeing to the doctors' relieving you of this part or that.

I still simply comply and try to joke with the young nurses who quiz me about my work, my college, my "perception" of my disease in a clumsy effort to get to know me better. I understand they are only following orders. As one explained, they want to know if I'm used to going to bed at 2:00 A.M. so they won't worry

33

if I wander the corridors in the wee hours. (Another asked a friend her religion. "None," she replied, and the nurse wrote down "Nun"). But last year when a resident who spurned my questions about the use of the word "total" instead of the expected "simple" to describe my forthcoming second mastectomy, then with an exasperated "I don't care!" tore up the consent form, I complained. The squeaky wheel gets the grease. Soon Tom Fahey was in my room explaining, "He's an anesthesiologist; he likes people better asleep than awake." (Hospitals now employ "patient representatives" if you need help in such a situation. Don't hesitate to call on them.)

There's another, brighter side of the coin. Almost everyone in the hospital tries, and you cannot help but respond. Talent abounds, and there are many well-trained professionals and, also important, paraprofessionals. Will I ever stop feeling grateful to the courtly attendant who wheeled me gently to the operating room, called me by my right name, checked my chart, and said a prayer for me for good measure? I particularly appreciated this because I had expected to be rolled, demerol-bleary to the operating room like a comatose beast. (A friend in this state had dimly heard an attendant ask if the breast about to be explored was the left. "*No*" she managed, "it's the right!" Another, in another hospital, fought to keep awake until her trusted surgeon's face swam into view, so frightened was she of the muddled confusion surrounding her.)

Nor will I forget the Sloan-Kettering radiology technicians, trained in transactional analysis, who rallied round me while I waited, crying, for a myelogram examination, "This is the place to cry, not in your room where you have to keep a stiff upper lip for your visitors." Then, skillfully, "Care to tell us what's the matter?" "All these awful things, and nothing seems to work." "Nothing seems to *work,* or nothing seems to *help*?" I cheered up; after all, I had been helped.

Fortunately for all of us, a strong trend now counteracts the mechanization of hospital life. There is a growing awareness in medical circles that we have lost too much to scientific speciali-

34

zation. There is an effort to look at you, the patient, as a whole human being, rather than a heart or lung or breast or set of bones. An example of this effort is a new system, in effect at many hospitals, notably Boston's Beth Israel, in which "primary nurses" are each assigned a few (perhaps four to six) patients. Instead of functioning as impersonal team specialists, dispensing medicines and often, if they are good, ending up in administrative jobs away from patients, they care for us from the time we enter the hospital through discharge, as "total people."

One nurse, in other words, is in charge of you throughout your hospital stay. She might visit you in the emergency room, in the recovery room, or intensive-care room before and after surgery. Nor is she above performing everyday routine chores for you in your hospital room, or answering phone call queries after you go home. Such a system really enables the staff to know you and care for you as an individual. It's being used increasingly, according to nurse consultant Marie Manthey, who has been going around the country tirelessly touting it.

Hooray! A nurse of my own would have avoided the sort of sadness I felt when I woke up in a hospitel room after my first mastectomy. I wanted to know what had happened to me. In pre-"two-stage" days, after my other biopsies, I had put my arm up to feel that the apparatus was still there, and it always was. This time I was too sick, too weak. Vomiting, I tried to raise my arm and failed. The face of the special recovery room nurse swam into sight. She was skilled and nice ("You don't feel well this morning, do you?"), but my surgeon was off performing his next operation, and I wanted to *know*. Finally, through the noisy buzz and the bright lights of the recovery room came the impersonal words: "She had a mastectomy."

If you are like most of the 952 patients and families interviewed in a study reported by Jerome Cohen of the UCLA School of Social Welfare, you will feel the time just after diagnosis as the most stressful; the period of hospitalization second, and the release from the hospital third. For me, it has been different. I feel cheerful in the hospital as the pain of surgery

35

wears off. The period when I return home to face everyday worries (Has the cat been fed? Is my job still there? Can I get someone to go to market for me?) and to confront my unbandaged self in the mirror ranks first, diagnosis second, and hospitalization last.

Indeed many patients relish the postsurgery parts of hospital life. Often the results of an intricate or even simple operation are excellent; the prognosis is too. Whatever the prognosis, nature helps you, secreting quantities of cortisone into your surgery-shocked body and leaving you hopeful and ebullient. Generally, you shake loose of the cares of job and household, to enjoy your visitors and the plants they bring (hospitals no longer encourage visitors to bring cut flowers, for they do not have enough vases and nurses do not have the time to arrange them).

Then too, both very social and very lonesome people often find solace and a sense of importance in the ministrations of the staff and the companionship of other patients. "I don't want to leave here," one such lonely, talkative lady on the picture-lined corridor of Sloan-Kettering's eighteenth floor confided. "If it weren't for the inconvenience of losing my breast, I'd say I'm having a good time here."

The ambience of these recuperative hospital days—"starched-white," with all that the term implies. On the one hand, it's a relief to have the operation over and done with and to be competently taken care of. On the other, you may worry about the injury done your body. Did the surgeon "get it all"? Will you be able to hide that scar on your face or arm behind makeup or clothes? Your colostomy left you feeling sort of dirty, having to run to the bathroom to empty that bag of waste; won't your friends find you "dirty" too? You may feel freakish, sexually repulsive with your lopsided breast or lost ovaries. Will anyone love you? Will you become hairy, like a man?

Don't think yourself odd if such questions nag you. The liaison psychiatrists, those who deal with the link between physical illness and the human condition, call them "basic threats to narcissistic integrity." For they undermine the sense that we are always capable and self-sufficient, that our bodies are indestructible, that we can control our own destiny. It's unlikely that you would discuss them with the phalanx of young residents and medical students who visit you on their morning rounds in a teaching hospital. They're too busy checking your heart with its vital sign readings (temperature, pulse, blood pressure) and thus your medical course, watching out for lapses, giving you another prod and poke, "That wound looks good. Anything we can do for you?"

You're lucky if you don't get one of the "sock it to 'em" remarks you may have heard at diagnosis, for they come most often from the "let-it-all-hang-out" generation in which residents are likely to fall: "Your rare cancer will certainly recur" ("Not so," said this young woman's doctor later; the young physician was just showing off his "knowledge"), or, to my friend, the late Vince Burke, a well-known foreign correspondent, "What *was* your profession, Mr. Burke?" When his wife, Vee, objected with, "What *is* his profession?", the doctor replied, "Well, you *are* an optimist."

No, you're not likely to discuss narcissistic threats with the residents. You're blessed if they just watch out for you, "What's this, still on a liquid diet two days after the operation?" Turning toward the nursing station, "Give her some scrambled eggs!"

It's different with the nurses. You see more of them than anyone else in the hospital. They give you "hands on" care, helping you perform your morning ablutions, checking on you routinely day and night, coming—it can be within minutes— when you buzz for them over the intercom ("May I help you?") Organized nursing talks a good deal about its "caring" function as opposed to the doctor's "curing" function, and I have indeed encountered many "caring" nurses. They give you answers at least to the first level of questions, telling you what's going to happen and how, "Your arm will be stiff for a few days after you go home, then it will gradually heal."

The problem is that with nurses in short supply, you often have a new nurse on every shift, every day. You will get the most support if you are lucky enough to have one of the new

37

breed of "primary care" nurses. She will really get to know you from the moment she comes in on your first day in the hospital with a cheery, "I'm your primary nurse. I'll be taking care of you while you're with us." You will also get support if you end up on a hospital floor where the "team" concept really works, where there is a real coming together of various caretakers around you, the patient.

In New York's Mount Sinai Hospital, and in some other hospitals too, the head nurse, primary oncologist, liaison psychiatrist, residents, and social worker conduct "Ombudsman rounds" every week on the cancer care unit. They talk about issues at a group meeting first, then interview the patient so he can express his feelings about his illness and his cure. Afterwards, the team discusses the patient's psychosocial problems and plans how to follow up to manage his care more effectively. Is he excessively active or passive? What drugs is he on? Why won't he do as he's advised? How is his family reacting to his disease? What can we do to help?

If there is a support group available to you or your family, like the one I attended last year at Sloan-Kettering, you'd be wise to take advantage of it. In this helpful Post-Mastectomy Rehabilitation group a nurse instructs you in hand and arm care and talks a little about the different prostheses, or falsies, on the market. A physical therapist takes you through a series of exercises to help you back to a normal range of motion: Your fingers climb the wall, reaching as far up as they are able, a bit more each day, or you bend over, swinging your arm loosely back and forth, or clasp your hands behind your neck and spread your wings. Then a social worker, helped by an attractive "Reach to Recovery" volunteer, leads you in a discussion of your concerns. The volunteer, a former patient herself, brings you your first downy temporary prosthesis and is good realistic proof that life can go on very nicely, postmastectomy.

Your family and friends can help greatly in this sort of supportive reassurance. Sometimes they do not know how to help or how to behave toward you (see chapter 6). For such people Sloan-Kettering psychiatrist Dr. Jimmie Holland has some good

38

advice. Interviewed for an in-house magazine along with hospital social workers, chaplains, and patient representatives, she stressed that generally it's important neither to ignore nor overemphasize the patient's disease when visiting him in the hospital. While most of us patients do not want to agonize over details, neither do we want friends to ignore the reality of our plight. Even if we look different, we are the same inside. We need to know we are still held in esteem and loved as before.

Specifically, the experts advised, visitors should not just drop in, they should knock before entering. They should greet you, the patient, as usual, with a kiss or a smile or a handshake.

They should not hover over you. They should sit close by you, and maintain eye contact with you. Instead of comparing your condition with what it was before, they should ask, "How are you feeling today?" or "How is your day going?"

Visitors should be good listeners, letting you take the lead in conversations. If you confide in them, they should listen and communicate openly. They should remember we patients do not want to talk about our diseases all the time. They should talk about themselves, their activities, and their interests—whether these be politics, fashion, sports, music, or news about mutual friends.

They should focus their visit on you, the patient, asking, "How can I help?" They should do things with you. Even in the hospital, they can usually take a walk with you or wheel you about. Outside, the world is their oyster.

Throughout, they should offer realistic support and reassurance, pointing out where help is available. They should pace their visits, planning some breaks. Knowing when to leave is important, in ten minutes, or an hour or two. They should simply say, "I think that I've stayed long enough." If you reply, "no," or "please stay," they should stay. If you agree, it is time for them to leave.

But it is the attending doctor in charge of your case who has the best chance of helping you now, mentally as well as physically. Unfortunately, he is often king in name only. He pops in for a few minutes, weekdays, on his rounds (or on his way to the golf course), leaving the real authority to the hospital with its chiefs of service, whom you do not see except in an emergency, and to the residents, who write the daily orders.

Still, in this postoperative period, your doctor can, and sometimes does, become the true "healing physician." He can, and sometimes does, become the "helper of the wounded, the encourager, the resolver of doubts," as Drs. Morton Bard and Arthur Sutherland have pointed out in a classic paper. ("Adaptation to Radical Mastectomy," which I read in the American Cancer Society's booklet, *The Psychological Impact of Cancer.*)

Help your doctor if he tries to capitalize on the rapport he established with you before the operation. Let him know that he is no longer the threatening superpower, with dreadful diagnosis and long knife, and that you expect his to be a healing mission. Give him cues that you want him to visit with you and if you wish, your family, in a relaxed way, and that you expect him not only to change dressings and examine your wound, but to chat casually and optimistically about your disease, your adjustment to surgery, and your future treatment.

This is particularly important if you are one of those patients who tends to get upset in the hospital, who "feels" a phantom limb or breast after an amputation or who wolfs food after a hysterectomy to fill up that gaping "hole." It's important even if you react more casually, outwardly euphoric but inwardly worrying about your weariness or poor appetite.

What you should expect is not someone who guarantees a cure or absolute relief from all your fears, but reassurance. You need someone you can trust, someone who will treat your disease with all the tools available, who will minimize its effects and keep you going as comfortably as possible. This usually means someone who stresses that you will retain a measure of independence, that you won't be a burden to your family, and that you will be accepted by other people, or, in a minority of cases, who will suggest you take your emotional aches and pains to a psychotherapist. And that someone is commonly your attending physician.

One woman complained after a brief surgical visit and curt outline of the treatment plan, "If only he'd just sat down a minute and talked a little." Another reported her oncologist talked to her honestly but tenderly and patiently. When she asked him if she was going to die, he responded that the doctors hoped the treatment would help her live a long time. He was "great" as opposed to her surgeon and a young resident who were of the "cancer is a fatal disease" school.

Perhaps these surgeons would have responded if the two women had spoken out plainly about their need for more of the doctor's time and informed understanding, "Look, I know you're a busy guy, but I need your help to explain where I am now and what's ahead. I've been too upset to absorb what you've told me so far. And my Cousin Susie has been telling me I should go to Europe and start xyz therapy, instead of what you suggest. Won't you have a seat and talk with me about all this?" Surgeons, often by nature "doers" who are more abruptly decisive and mechanically oriented than doctors in specialities where there is more time for reflection, sometimes need a little prod like this.

So might those other doctors who develop an abrupt, aloof, uncaring mask to protect themselves from pain but underneath care very much about what's happening to you. If you try to let such a physician know your needs but still feel that you cannot talk openly and comfortably with him, and so trust him, it might be best for both of you to seek referral to someone else (easier, of course, in a big city than a small one, but still possible if you switch from surgeon to radiologist or medical oncologist or back to your personal physician as your main source of care). For right now, you need real support.

You need this support especially because this is decision-making time. The decision-making process, which starts in the doctor's office and may continue intermittently for many years, reaches its peak in the hospital as your medical caretakers assess your condition and map out your treatment plan.

All hanging-in patients face some decisions, but cancer

41

patients sometimes feel as though choices are exploding all around them. For example, your doctors may feel you need radiation therapy, the use of high energy rays to stop cancer cells from growing and multiplying. When you first see the radiologist, he draws lines or tatoo marks precisely around the area where your cancer is located, then computes the exact dosage of "rads" (radiation absorbed dose) you will need.

For several weeks you will be left alone for a few minutes each day in a sort of bulletproof room with a giant machine (mine was a linear accelerator) whose rays attack all the cells within their reach and destroy the more sensitive cancer cells' ability to reproduce. In the newer internal radiation therapy, small amounts of radioactive material or implants are placed inside your body, or directly on the cancer, and left there for a period of time.

You may need chemotherapy, usually intravenous treatment with drugs powerful enough to poison the cancer cells in your body. When I first had cancer, doctors gave chemotherapy only when the cancer had spread widely. Now they give "adjuvant" chemotherapy to patients with early stages of cancer, to prevent its spreading.

Chemotherapists or oncologists usually mix their own chemotherapy "cocktails." They feel there's safety in numbers; if one does not work, another will. Alkylating agents, like cytoxan, stop or slow down cell growth. Antimetabolites, 5-Fluorouracil (5 FU) for instance, mimic normal nutrients so that they are taken up by the cancer cell; once inside they interfere with the dividing process and prevent cell growth. Antibiotics made from soil fungi, like Adriamycin, block cell growth. Chemicals from the periwinkle plant, vincristine, for one, interfere with cell division.

And you may need hormone therapy to manipulate your body's hormonal balance and challenge cancerous cells. This is necessary especially for those breast cancer patients whose estrogen receptor assay tests have proved positive. The purpose of this laboratory test, which should be done routinely on all malignant breast tissue after it is diagnosed, is to see whether parts of your cancer cells can be bound to estrogen molecules. If they can be so bound, you would benefit, like me, either from surgery to remove your estrogen-producing ovaries (oöphorectomy or ovariectomy) and/or some type of antiestrogen drug, such as Tamoxifen, which affects the estrogens produced by your glands. Such drugs are taking the place of drastic operations to remove the adrenal gland or message-sending pituitary gland.

You may need some combination of all these therapies, as I have. You may need more. You may elect to have reconstructive mammoplasty. This means you have the surgeons implant an artificial breast made of silicone under your skin sometime after your original surgery. They can even make a new nipple for you, or preserve your original one! A third of Sloan-Kettering breast chief Dr. David Kinne's patients are having such reconstruction now. You will have to discuss all these things with your doctor.

The options have to be laid out for you, the pros and cons listed. At Boston's Women's-Brigham Hospital, I listened as Dr. Barbara McNeil told me about a new form of decision making that factors patient attitudes into medical decisions. Using *decision analysis*, an industrial technique, doctors consider every possible outcome of every course of action. They assign a numerical *probability* to the likelihood of that outcome's occurrence. After interviewing the patient in depth, they assign a numerical *utility*, which reflects the relative worth of the outcome. The sum of the probability and utility for every potential consequence of a therapeutic choice is the *expected value* of that therapy.

The rational decision maker can then select the therapy with the greatest expected value. Thus, in one study, patients with "operable" lung cancer were interviewed about their feelings as to surgery versus radiation. The doctors found many patients quite averse to taking the risk of the possibility of immediate death involved in surgery. When their attitudes were combined with data about survival after both therapies, it appeared that radiotherapy was the preferred form of treatment for several patients.

However, Dr. Randall Cebul, the University of Pennsylvania professor who heads the recently founded Society for Medical Decision Making, points out that though patient attitudes must be considered, some patients do not *want* to submit to the cold hard question interviewing process. Doctors must alert students and others to the need to be sensitive to patients' feelings.

I agree. It seems to come back to this: You need a physician who will listen patiently to you, answering your questions with candor but compassion, as positively as possible, and taking cues from you as to what you want to know, when, and how. You may be a patient who wants to know everything and participate in every single decision about your illness. Or you may feel more at ease leaving matters for the most part in your doctor's hands. Or you may want to make decisions slowly, in stages, one day, one week at a time, rather than all at once.

However you feel, it is important that you know your treatment plan and feel comfortable with it. Only then can you feel as though you are a cooperating team player, fighting your disease. Physician "honesty" should be evaluated, as Dr. Mark Lipkin suggested in a *Newsweek* "My Turn" column, not only in terms of a slavish devotion to language you might misinterpret, but also in terms of intent. In other words, the goal of the dialogues between you, the patient, and your doctor, should be to benefit *you*. It's that simple.

One must add that the decision-making process is complicated by the fact that new therapies are being tested all the time. For example, we patients might read about the new immunotherapy drug Interferon, in a *Time* magazine cover story, only to find our hopes extinguished when we ask our doctors excitedly if it is for us, "I don't think so," one told me, "we've used it with some success in some patients, but it has been a disappointment in breast and many other cancers."

A Johns Hopkins cancer specialist observed, "There are no secrets in this business," and he's right. "If they knew what to do they'd all be doing it," another commented. Discoveries are usually a long time coming, and when, like the polio vaccine, they prove effective, it's hard to withhold them. By the time you read this, a new one may have become an established reality. The last time I was at Sloan-Kettering, Tom Fahey seemed, for the first time, genuinely excited about such an embryonic treatment: therapy with hybridomas. In the new hybridoma technology, the durable qualities of the cancer cell are combined with the disease-fighting properties of the body's own antibodies to fight specific cancers.

Added to all the complexities of the traditional therapies, we now have the so-called nontraditional ones. Patients usually arrive at such therapies later, after the more conventinal ones become more ineffective (or more painful and exhausting). These unproven therapies may be drugs, like Laetrile or Krebiozen (now discredited after scientific clinical trials) or coffee enema-type approaches which flourish south of the border in Mexico, or the "holistic" treatments that cover a mishmash of treatments from acupuncture to imagery.

But I came to all this later in my journey.

Chapter 4

A NEW SUBCULTURE: THE NOT QUITE WELL

The Karnofsky Performance Chart hung on the chemotherapy clinic bulletin board until I reported on it in *The Washington Post.* Then, "they," the patients' designation for the medical establishment, understood its threatening nuances for us and removed it.

But it still appears on the lower-right-hand corner of the Oncology Flow Chart on which the doctors mark my progress, or lack of it. I measure somewhere between 80 percent on good days *(Able to carry on normal activities with effort)* and 70 percent on bad ones *(Unable to carry on normal activities but cares for self).* I can slip to 60 percent *(Requires occasional assistance with personal needs)* if "personal needs" means not brushing my teeth, but driving the car or shopping.

It could be better: 100 percent *(Normal)* or 90 percent *(Minor signs or symptoms).* It could be worse: 50 percent *(Receives considerable assistance and medical care);* 40 percent *(Disabled);* 30 percent *(Severely disabled and hospitalized);* 20 percent *(Very sick, active supportive treatment necessary);* or even 10 percent *(Moribund).*

"Where's zero?" I asked, when I first saw the chart. It was a half joke. I had been familiar with the way doctors "stage" cancer patients, according to the distance the tumor travels in the body. If you are in stage one, the tumor is limited to the organ in which it originated; if you are in stage four, it has spread to remote organs and nodes. That had been medical gobbledygook. The more mundane Karnofsky Performance Chart made me finally realize I had become part of a new cancer subculture, the subculture of the hanging-in patient.

I am not moribund. I am not usually in the hospital. But I am—face it—not quite well. A sword of Damocles hangs over my head. Like most swords of Damocles, it feels uncomfortable. "Where have you been?" asks the tailor, when I go to pick up my coat in late November, instead of mid-September. "Listen," I tell him, "you're lucky I'm here at all." When the printer asks me if I want 500 or 1,000 sheets of business stationery for the free-lance writing enterprise I am restarting, I hesitate. "One thousand is a bargain," he advises, "but a bargain isn't a bargain if you don't use it." I grin. But I pick 500.

Some doctors are successful with hanging-in patients for whom they prescribe a "normal" life. If patients interpret this admonition simply as doing as much as they comfortably can and forgetting the rest, they have no trouble with it. I've noticed leukemia patients, particularly, tend to feel well when they are in remission and act accordingly. When asked how it feels to have leukemia, Robert Fisher, a long-time Sloan-Kettering patient and volunteer worker, answered, "I'd rather have a Danish." Then he bicycled across the country to dispel the notion that cancer is a constant problem. "I can't pretend to feel anything but fine," he told reporters.

What an enviable state! I am living my life, but it is, as a public television show I appeared in was titled, "A Different Kind of Life." I have to force myself to ask my young colleague at the Department of Education secretariat, Fred Register, to please feed the parking meter for me and get the cokes while we are working. I have to admit I sometimes miss the cane I used for a short time after radiation to my hip. This is true especially on a crowded bus or subway when no one thinks to offer me a seat. The wicker seatback I carry around to meetings obviously fails to send out adequate signals.

I ride up and down on the therapy roller coaster, up and about, down and out. I have to pace myself. I have to leave crowded stifling stand-up parties when my back acts up and I can't find an empty chair. (Since my vertebra collapsed in 1977 I have lived with a permanent slipped disc.) I have to identify the things I want to do—planting the geraniums, reading Jane Austen, traveling to Haiti with Tina Fredericks, my old friend, trying to assemble my thoughts compellingly on paper. I have to separate them from the things that mean less to me, do them, and let the others go.

No, my life, as you know if you are a hanging-in patient, is not normal. Whether you suffer cancer or another chronic disease, your life is "different." It is a life in which I worry how my wig and my falsies appear, a world where I spend hours, too many hours, visiting doctors and their clinics. It is a world where I trade precious time for treatment and risk treatment for precious time. This treatment has its own ambience, changing, but alas, never ending. I do not hate it because I look on it as a sort of protective shield in my battle against those ugly, aggressive cancer cells.

Treatment is my powerful ally, but not a completely trustworthy one, for it saps my strength and creates its own problems. I was a consultant to a conference on health policy held at a motel near Dulles Airport when I started my radiation course, after the cancer metastasized to my spine in 1977. I remember I had forced myself out there although I felt slightly woozy.

Once at the conference, my throat tightened; I could not swallow dinner. I went to my room, lay down on the narrow bed, felt the world sway, and reached over weakly to call my husband to come and get me. Then I tried to call the radiologists. While I hung onto the phone, waiting, I wondered if the high energy rays emitted by that formidable metal x-ray machine had destroyed a few cells too many along my spine, and if the young

49

technicians handling it knew what they were doing. But the doctor reassured me; it was nothing to worry about, a normal reaction; I should take another Atarax pill (tranquilizer). My husband called for me. Back home, I went to bed and slept for eighteen hours straight.

I haven't slept so much since, though I've sometimes felt like it. I grew used to that horrendous treatment. Soon it was routine to make my daily trip to the hospital waiting room, with its cheery orange walls, change from street clothes to my green hospital gown, and lie on a cot alone with my friend the linear accelerator, monitored through closed-circuit TV by a technician outside the treatment room. Two years later when the cancer in my hip was radiated, I felt nothing but slight weariness.

Not so with the chemotherapy, which came a few months later, after the disease spread further through my bones. I wept on and off for a week when I started my chemo course, so afraid was I of the nausea, weariness, and God knows what other symptoms it might create. But they did not turn out as hard for me as for some patients, and, of course, they are a low price to pay for these extra years of life. But they *do* persist, rearing their less-than-charming heads the day after I return from the George Washington University Medical Center clinic. When the effects of the compazine shot the nurse gives me and suppository I take at night wear off, it's whoopsing time.

Positives: Neither the chemotherapy treatment nor its side effects last long. I only have to endure it twice a month. My hair has grown back after two years of semibaldness. It's short and not as thick as it was, but it's there. And though my voice sank an octave or two after a period of hormone therapy (with halotestin, a male hormone), people say it now sounds better than my sister's. Nothing else changed. I did *not* grow a beard.

Caveat: Hospital boards and administrators should be more aware of the effect hanging-in patients' surroundings have on their progress. They've blessed me and other oncology-hematology outpatients at George Washington with a competent, empathetic group of nurses, headed by nurse-practitioner

Peg Lloyd (who once, to save me an elevator ride, came down to the street and drew blood from my arm as I sat in my parked car: "Curbside therapy" she observed).

But the tiny treatment room the nurses must use is depressing, with its two reclining lounge chairs separated by a green curtain from two somber, black armchairs. When all of these are filled with what one friend called "shades" (very ill, very gaunt, vomiting sufferers), taking their chemotherapy from a wilderness of hanging bottles and tubes, or with sickle-cell anemia patients in painful, pitiful crisis, it's hard to stay upbeat. Put yourself in our place, powers that be! Even though money is short and resources scarce, try to give us all, nurses and patients, some space, some privacy.

In an anonymous government pamphlet, of all places, *Coping with Cancer: A Resource for the Health Professional*, I came across a way of looking at the general issues confronting cancer patients. I liked it and traced it to its source. She is Mila Tecala, a bright, cheerful clinical social worker, who took a job working with cancer patients years ago at Georgetown University Medical Center because no one else wanted it (she says). Now she practices on her own in a homey Massachusetts Avenue office in Northwest Washington, D.C. Like many therapists I've met who see cancer patients primarily, she loves her work. She finds it "very satisfying," much more meaningful than an ordinary my-husband-won't-help-with-the-dishes practice. She is hooked.

I challenged her while we chatted in her big comfortable armchairs, not about the content, but about the arrangement of the four issues she had identified as concerning cancer patients: *alienation, mutilation, mortality, vulnerability*. I said mutilation comes first, then alienation, then vulnerability (loss of control). Mortality comes last, but is ever present.

Mila Tecala agreed. Certainly *mutilation*—the results of what one of her patients called "cutting, burning, and poisoning"— comes first. Surgery, radiation, and chemotherapy, the widely used "conventional" treatments, leave many patients de-

51

pressed. Losing a functioning integral part of you, a bladder, a womb, a lung, can be saddening. Losing a more visible breast or eye or leg can be traumatic. Such a lost body part may be perceived as part of a happier life, synonymous with wholeness, with belonging, with activity, with being worthwhile. You grieve for them when they are gone. As you grieve you may have trouble sleeping or eating. Why can't you concentrate? Fearing rejection, you may withdraw from life—from work, from social and sexual relations.

I cried a lot at first, even after I left the hospital. But I have grown accustomed to mutilation as I have gone along. In an overwhelmingly breast-conscious society, a society where the big tit epitomizes big femininity, even small attractiveness, I asked, "Why me?" I was glad prostheses (false breasts) were available, but I had a hard time getting used to the idea of wearing them. It took me several trips to a local department store to find one just the right size and shape. (Much later, I discovered an even better one with a nipple at a New York mastectomy boutique, and later still, when I needed two, I bought improved lightweight, and smaller, ones). Some people, like my friend Peggy, never do find a suitable falsie to help them lose that lopsided look and feeling. A decade after surgery, she still stuffs her bra with an old stocking.

Six and a half years later, when I had a second mastectomy to remove a breast afflicted by a completely different, rare cancer, I felt very different, almost numb. The operation seemed a simple exchange: another lovely part for another lovely piece of life. Perhaps my extensive treatment has left me more understanding and so less fearful. I know what's coming.

If Alice Roosevelt Longworth could wisecrack about her predicament as a "topless nonagerian," why couldn't I? Mila Tecala laughs often as she talks. She stresses the importance of maintaining your sense of humor. So do many people. If you succeed, like Hubert Humphrey during his long treatment for cancer, you are blessed. Senator Humphrey often pointed out that if you start taking yourself too seriously, you lose perspective. In the Virgin Islands, he liked to tell friends, "What a wonderful place this is! They've got Greta Garbo who doesn't talk to anybody and Hubert Humphrey who'll talk to everybody."

Others have trouble laughing at themselves. If you feel you do not like your mutilated self, how can you expect other people to like you?

Such patients feel *alienated*, alone. In the rawest circumstances, a grandmother will not let her granddaughters see their hospitalized mother because she believes cancer to be contagious. In a less brutal, but still hurtful, way a cherished cousin stays away because in his mind cancer means death and he cannot bring himself to face the idea of death. Most of my friends are more sophisticated and sensitive than this. But some have certainly alienated me. They may admire the way I "cope," but they consider me special, different from themselves, to be put in a separate, secret folder on a shelf (more of that later, in chapter 6).

Social worker Tecala talks about "mutual alienation." She says families, overwhelmed by a father or son's cancer, can overwhelm him. They mourn his loss before it occurs. They hover about him, making him feel more helpless and hopeless than he needs to feel. They say, "You're OK," when that's not true, and he responds, "I'm OK," whether he feels he is or not. Honest communication fails, and that failure snowballs.

Such a failure may have been acceptable when a diagnosis often meant three months of life. But now, doctors talk not only in terms of "remission" but in terms of "cure." They speak of a "normal life span." Patients cannot risk alienation from their families and close friends for eight or ten or twenty years. Sensing this, we may test to see who alienates us. Teenagers do this especially well. They say: "Hey, how do you like my bald head? I'm Kojak!" Showing off their wounds, they send a clear message, "Here I am. Take me. Accept me, or leave me."

I can understand the flashing of such badges of courage. I flash mine sometimes too. By being candid and open about my illness and its results, I try to show others I am strong, in control, independent. I try to show myself I am not *vulnerable*.

Mila Tecala reports that in her native Philippines, dependency is acceptable to a degree. No one raises an eyebrow when a thirty- to forty-year-old bachelor lives with his parents, or when elderly grandparents stay with their children and grandchildren. But here in the United States, you have to be self-sufficient, by golly. You have to be independent. You cannot lose autonomy or the right to govern your own life.

Such a culture is particularly hard on hanging-in patients. It tells us to act strong and certain. Yet we live with uncertainty. We do not know how long our disease will last or how it will affect us. Heart patients can control their disease by taking their medicines regularly, or dieting, or exercising in a special way. By contrast, there often seems to be little we can do to control cancer's onslaught. No wonder *they* are heart "patients," while *we* are cancer "victims."

I feel this keenly, for I am by nature an independent person. I glory when there is something I can "do" about my disease, like arranging a medical consultation, or buying a brace, or even having an operation to remove a cancerous breast or estrogen-secreting ovary. I suffer when my legs are weak and I cannot drive a car. I bark at my husband when he is nice enough to drive me on errands. I anguish when I have to acquire a chair glide to carry me up and down the back stairs because my hips and legs hurt too much to climb them on my own. I sympathize with my friend and fellow hanging-in patient Diana when she calls me with "Great News!" Did her doctor find her a cure? No, but she had a real bowel movement on her own (no enema).

I try as hard as I can to control pain when I suffer it. Pain is a slippery subject for us hanging-in patients. It comes and goes, waxes and wanes. It is demoralizing, hard to describe to our caretakers, hard for them to pin down. And, doctors tell me, it is still handled by many of them in a haphazard, inadequate way.

Actually, there are two kinds of pain. Acute pain is easy. It has a beginning, suffered after a fracture, for instance, or a surgical incision. It has a middle, usually treatment with analgesic drugs. It has an end, which comes with healing. Almost everyone has suffered it at times; almost everyone empathizes with it.

Chronic pain is a different story. It lasts and lasts, displaying

54

neither rhyme nor reason. It can eat you up, consuming all your time and attention, keeping you from work or school or just plain fun, and depressing you (which in turn accelerates the pain and leaves you vulnerable to more). It can come from the disease itself as it did when cancer attacked my spine and my vertebra collapsed or when my sister's arthritis flared up in her bones. Or it can be secondary to the primary disease itself, coming from a urinary tract infection that weakened blood cells have trouble fighting, or from something completely different, like a sinus-induced, splitting headache.

At Sloan-Kettering, a special pain clinic addresses cancer pain. The pain team working there realizes the importance of analgesics (like Tylenol or aspirin) taken regularly and in adequate doses, before the effect of the previous dose has worn off. This team does not fear, as do too many physicians, the use of narcotic analgesics, morphine and the like. Discharged outpatients on large oral doses have not used these drugs illegally, have not attempted suicide, and have withdrawn from them without major problems.

What's more, the Sloan-Kettering pain experts are studying new ways of attacking pain: neurosurgically, by blocking certain pathways to the brain; psychotherapeutically, through antianxiety or antidepressant medication or through such techniques as hypnosis. They are deeply interested in recent discoveries of the opiate receptor in the brain, believed to be the neurotransmitter of natural as well as administered analgesics, and of the brain's endorphins, substances believed to have analgesic properties similar to morphine.

Therapists in other places too are beginning to use all available weapons to help cancer patients fight pain. One of the new ones used by Drs. Stephen Hersh and Lucy Waletzky in their Medical Illness Counseling Center is transcutaneous electrical nerve stimulation (TENS), in which tiny wires placed on your skin interrupt the pain waves. This all-out antipain approach is the one I seek now, instead of the more dated "as little as possible" one personified by the Washington, D.C. doctor who was shocked at the Levo-Dromoran prescribed for me at Sloan-Kettering after an operation. "It's the first cousin to morphine!"

he exclaimed. I assured him I would *not* become a drug addict. "Any one can," he answered, and I knew he included doctors. The bottle is still on my shelf, three-quarters full.

So it goes. I do the crossword puzzle in the morning paper each day to prove to myself that my brain is still working. I rented the chair glide for six months, then I either had to buy it or turn it back. I no longer needed it, but I was afraid to turn it back. This was because of the fourth, over-reaching issue confronting cancer patients: *mortality.*

"Death is my friend," said Thalia, a patient in a cancer support group I attended at George Washington University Hospital, "I play hide and seek with him." She has outwitted him for thirty years, she told me. She is comfortable with him.

I am not, at least, not yet. He is not my friend, he is my enemy, still to be fought and kept at bay. Yet like Thalia, I have to live with him, over there in that dark cloud on the horizon, in the background music of each day. I'm about to rewrite my will again and to go over the list in which I assign my favorite trinkets to favorite friends. I gloried in my son Jeremy's recent wedding, I was able to *be there!*

I try to avoid the medical mighties who with their harsh "honest" words—and I cannot say it often enough—deprive me of the hope that I can fend off my enemy, death. I understand why a Virginia oncologist decided never again to tell patients "honestly" that death is imminent after a man she socked it to in this way retreated dramatically into depression and Valium. I am still peeved at the physician who told me over the telephone when my second breast cancer was diagnosed, "We have to stop talking in terms of cure and begin talking in terms of control—one year, maybe two." Dr. Tom Fahey commented, "How does he know?"

He does not know. "Don't worry, dearie," said a cheerful Irish lady, a fellow cancer patient in the x-ray department, who was walking around with all sorts of tubes attached to her, "The Lord won't take you any sooner than he intended."

It was a comforting thought.

CHAPTER 5

TOOLS AND CRUTCHES

Harry, the blind jogger. I met him where I least expected, in a film shown at the annual conference of Washington's St. Francis Society (which deals with the problems of life-threatening illness). In the film, he ran a race, yoked arm-and-arm to an anonymous fellow runner.

Both were men of indeterminate young age. Both wore conventional jogging outfits. Harry wore a sign saying, "Blind man." Both concentrated intensely on the race. As they threaded their way through a beautiful but twisted trail, they discussed the pitfalls confronting them. No rock or boulder or thorny branch escaped their analysis. They planned their strategy ("We're splitting from the rest").

Dr. Charles A. Garfield led the discussion following the film at this conference, the theme of which was "The Psychology of Survival." A tousled-haired University of California, San Francisco, psychologist, he founded and heads the SHANTI project in which some 350 volunteers have served over 2,000 patients with life-threatening illness. What is real help, he asked an audience composed largely of counselors and therapists whose daily job is to give it. What energies, what "coping styles," can be used to help a fellow human being, blind or ill?

Harry had electrified the audience. So had his nameless helper, for obviously Harry could not have run the race alone. Even his blunt sign, "Blind Man," was not enough. He needed the eyes his yoked partner shared with him to maneuver the trail. More, he needed the sense of mission they shared—the will to run, to take risks, perhaps even to win the race. He needed to trust his partner, and he needed his partner's trust in his own ability to make it, much more than pity for the fact that, unseeing, he might stumble and fall by the wayside.

Like Harry, every hanging-in patient needs help in dealing with the mighty issues confronting her, or him. As California oncologist Dr. Ernest Rosenbaum puts it, we need "tools and crutches." I do not care who you are, or how much money, or status, or inner strength you can muster. You need help.

When I was first sick with cancer, a world ago now, it was not easy to find such help. "Should I go to a psychiatrist?" I asked my surgeon, Dr. Calvin Klopp, when we discussed my postmastectomy blues. "If you know one you have a relationship with, that would be wonderful," replied this senior physician in a city with one of the highest ratios of psychiatrists to patients in the country. "But I do not know any I want to recommend. I knew just one who was good with cancer patients, but he moved away."

Dr. Klopp is retired now, but he was a competent, humane specialist in "North of the Border" cancer (of the chest, neck, head, and skin). What he was telling me, I think, was that in his broad experience, conventional help tended to force patients to face reality, and reality might not be all that therapeutic. But I persisted, asking if I could contact a *"Reach to Recovery"* support volunteer for breast cancer patients. Again he shook his head. "If I could screen all the volunteers, it would be all right," he told me. "But I cannot, and I've seen too many of them hanging up the crepe."

How times have changed! If you are a patient with chronic illness now, you can choose from a host of helpers. You can find such helpers in "support groups" based at hospitals or out in the community (self-help or therapy groups of patients and their

58

families, concerned with the same disease, led by health professionals). You can find such helpers among the many highly trained individual counselors like Mila Tecala, be he or she a social worker, nurse, psychiatrist, psychologist, clergyman, or volunteer.

With optimistic, resourceful, realistic help, you can gather the information you need, analyze and come to understand it, then you can get a handle on whatever you fear, keep your balance, regain your sense of self-worth and self-esteem. With such help you can sort out your options and figure out how you can spend your time most meaningfully.

With such help you can, as the psychiatrists put it, "cope." At one time I did not like to use the word *cope,* a holdover from my days as an assistant to Connecticut's Senator Abraham Ribicoff. ("Don't use the word *cope,*" he once told me. "People who sit on the floor say *cope.*") But now, in the days of a whole *coping* literature, I know no other word that will fill the bill. In fact, psychiatrist Dr. Avery Weisman points out in his fine booklet, *Coping With Cancer,* there is a dimension beyond diagnosis, treatment, and relief called "safe conduct." This means how to conduct you, the patient, through the hanging-in maze, in all seasons and states, through thick and thin. And this, in turn, means how to help you "cope."

Weisman, a Harvard Medical School Professor of Psychiatry who directs the Omega research project at Massachusetts General Hospital, feels the coping process combines several different kinds of strategies. These are both active and passive, depending on the purpose, and vary from seeking more information (rational inquiry) and sharing concern and talk with others (mutuality), to trying to forget; putting your dilemma out of your mind (suppression) or blaming someone or something else (externalize, project). No strategy works for all your problems, whether it be laughing it off (affect reversal), or doing other things for distraction (displacement/redirection).

Some work better and more often than others. Denial, which revises or reinterprets a portion of the painful reality you face, is a phase of the coping process. It is, as one doctor put it, the

59

"morphine of the soul," and it can help as well as hinder, avoiding what threatens in the future, and holding fast to what is helpful in the past.

No help can bring the hanging-in patient everlasting equanimity. Few people achieve that. But effective help can bring your distress within tolerable limits. It can aid in managing your principal problems.

Of course, not everyone can take advantage of such help. Some disdain it altogether. Others, like a hospital roommate I once had, prefer to rely completely on their doctors. "If I had a problem," she told me, "I'd take it to my doctor. That social worker is too nosey." But I have grown more lucky at getting substantial help and more savvy about what I need, and when. Very early on, I was wary of support groups whose members might intrude on my privacy or burden me with still heavier problems than my own.

I was wary, too, of therapists who might try some weird way of laying hands on me. I consulted a traditional psychiatrist, but one flexible enough to talk as well as listen, even to make suggestions and visit me in the hospital. He helped me particularly with close-to-the-heart problems—my family who loved me but tried to overprotect me, or my colleagues who could not quite take my candor about my cancer, or the work I longed to do but could not muster the strength to tackle.

Then, in the middle of a dark hospital night after my cancer had begun to spread widely a nurse caught me crying in my bed at Sloan-Kettering. She asked me what was the matter, and when I grunted, "Nothing," she suggested that I see Sister Rosemary Moynihan, the social worker on the twelfth floor. I argued, "I've been through all that. I've seen a psychiatrist. I don't need any Sister Rosemary."

But I hurt, and finally I allowed as how I'd see the good sister, once. I saw her the next morning and still see her whenever I get the chance. At first I could not look at her without weeping. She helped me see that I wept because I was for the first time recognizing—mourning, as it were, the progress of my disease.

60

After awhile, I was able to discuss calmly with her the radioactive rays chasing the cancer around my body or the poisons about to be poured into my system. "Adriamycin," she told me, "is called the red devil," and we talked about what help I might get if this devil made me nauseous.

Like other social workers, Sister Rosemary acted as a sort of liaison for me with the strange new hanging-in subculture I was entering. She helped me integrate the odd new world of platelets and prostheses into my own life and helped me feel safer in dealing with it. Using her considerable skill at pumping the telephone to find out what agencies and programs produce what services and at what cost, she moved into my life in a practical way. She found me a comfortable, moderately-priced temporary apartment in housing near Sloan-Kettering. My husband and children could visit me and help me while I completed my radiation course. I could walk to the outpatient clinic for treatment.

Back home in Washington, D.C., some months later, I found a support group at George Washington University Medical Center. Led jointly by a psychiatric nurse and a social worker, as are most such groups (two leaders help each other pick up verbal and nonverbal cues from patients), it met weekly at the hospital for a discussion of mutual concerns. Some problems they helped us air seemed horrendous at first: Why take on the loss of a testicular cancer patient's balls when I had enough handling my lost bosom? But I came to look at the group's concerns differently. The heavier they were, the more ordinary mine seemed. As one elderly gentleman put it, "I felt sorry for myself because I had no shoes until I met a man who had no feet." Eventually I got a real lift when two patients who had been through bilateral cancer surgery told me how much more balanced and comfortable I would feel after my second mastectomy.

It is amazing how that gnawing feeling in your stomach goes away when other patients tell you some of their friends avoid them too; it's not just miserable old you. Or that they, too, had to tell a mother or an aunt please not to call every minute to ask how they were doing. Hospital-based groups can be organized around disease sites (colo-rectal or breast) or treatment mode (radiotherapy or rehabilitation) or patient age. At Sloan-Kettering, with its more than 500 cancer patients, there is a social worker on every floor and a multitude of groups of post-surgical breast, or presurgical thoracic patients, of children with leukemia and their families and doctors, of families of the seriously ill.

Out in the community, too, there are a variety of groups for colostomy, mastectomy, and laryngectomy patients (I like the name of the latter in Washington, the "Lost Chord Club"). Some, like "CanSurmount" and "Reach to Recovery," send selected and trained volunteers to visit with other cancer patients; others, such as "I Can Cope" or "Make To-day Count," have developed educational and psychological programs to suit various needs.

Of course, not all patients are comfortable in groups. They may be shy, private people, who for one reason or another feel they would benefit more from one-to-one counseling. Individual therapists and counselors trained to work with such hanging-in patients abound. They listen to your words and observe your body language, creating a nonjudgmental atmosphere that gives you the freedom to express your innermost anxieties and concerns. As we hang in longer and longer the "helping professions" have turned their attention from helping us toward a death with dignity to helping us toward a life of quality. It's heartening when after a counseling session you can decide to be selfish, in a sense, after a lifetime of "Après vous, Alphonse," and do what works for you, whether it's little or big, buying that extra wicker seatback from Hammacher Schlemmer, or taking that part-time job at the Department of Education, or conserving your energy by declining an invitation.

A caveat, friend hanging-in patient: Be scrupulous in checking out the credentials of those who offer you their services, whether they be as individual therapists or group leaders. This is not a time when you can afford to fall into the hands of poorly trained people who take advantage of your vulnerability.

A friend of a friend wrote to tell me she lived in Fair Haven, New Jersey, and could not find a suitable support group to help her while she hung in there with cancer. What to do? I advised her to find the number of the nearest American Cancer Society Division (there is at least one in every state) and ask for the services person who could direct her to an individual counselor, or whatever kind of patient group she wanted—based in a hospital or the community, composed of patients and families, or just patients, or stressing contact between patients and volunteers (who are usually seasoned cancer patients themselves).

The central American Cancer Society office in New York (212-371-2900) would have that number if she couldn't find it locally, and so would the Cancer Information Service (CIS), a national network of toll-free telephone lines run by the federal government's research center, the National Cancer Institute. The national CIS number is 800-638-6694; some states also have a Cancer Information Service, and most CIS offices are associated with Comprehensive Cancer Centers. Breast Cancer patients might want to consult consumerist Rose Kushner's advisory service (Box 224, Kensington, MD 20795), though she is better known for pretreatment counseling, especially her advocacy of the two-stage mastectomy.

Parents of children with cancer would surely want to get in touch with Candlelighters, an active and constructive group offering a variety of services. And there are groups for many other types of hanging-in patients and their families. I just heard of a Pennsylvania hospital group for families of heart attack patients. There a spouse or child can gather hints about what a cardiac patient should eat or how much exercise he should get, as well as how to help him emotionally.

I had discarded my clumsy back brace, which made me sweat, and my clothes balloon. But nagging back pain still kept me constant company. Doctors and the Sloan-Kettering pain clinic had only given me more pills. Small doses of Elavil, the latest pain killer, had made my hands tremble.

I wanted competent, not shaky hands. Seeking new help, I consulted a psychologist, Lester Turner, who specializes in hypnosis and pain control. I had read about hypnosis; I knew a hypnotic state is an altered state of mind or consciousness. I knew that in such a state I could suspend some of the functions of my conscious, wakeful mind and focus my attention on a few inner realities. I could become more receptive than usual to suggestions or direction.

This psychologist had helped my friend Nick Kotz give up smoking; he had helped others stop overeating. Could he help me dull my pain? Would I lose control over my mind? Terrified, I sat in his office armchair, listening to his soft voice, "Natalie, find a comfortable position. Find something to focus your attention on. I'm going to count from one to three. At one, I want you to do one thing, at two, two things, at three, three things. . . ."

This was not so bad, after all, "First take a deep breath and hold it. Breathe in relaxation, breathe out tension." The hypnotic tapes Les gave me to practice with at home did not wipe away my pain. Using one, called "glove anesthesia," I could put my hand to sleep by thinking about the last time the dentist gave me Novocain. But I could not, even in a trance-like state, transfer the numbness to my aching back. Nor could I, using another tape, forget that aching back completely by returning to the past and focusing my full attention on a Washington Press Club trip I had taken to Russia some years before.

Still, the tapes did help me relax my tense muscles, and, in so doing, they helped make me more open to a different kind of thinking about the mind-body connection, whose adherents had been bombarding me, as a medical writer, with leaflets and brochures advertising their wares: "Holistic Health: Family Practice of the 80s"; "The Psychology of Survival"; "Moshe Feldenkrais' Awareness Through Movement"; "Guided Imagery as a Therapeutic Technique"; "Workshop on Therapeutic Touch"; "Getting Well Again—One Team's Approach to Healing Cancer and Improving Health." Originating in the Ancient

East, renewed under the tolerant skies of sunny California, Holism had obviously exploded in my own darker, more skeptical Northeast.

If so many people, some of them seemingly respectable, were involved in holistic practices, might there not be something to them, at least to the psychological approaches? During my repeated bouts with cancer, the wild holistic mix of bodily, social, and psychological interventions—meditation, acupuncture, yoga, biofeedback, imagery—had seemed for the birds, or at least for the young, prevention-minded, veggie-consuming counterculturist, not for a middle-aged cancer patient like me, whose grandmother had gotten cancer at just about the same age, and in the same pattern.

What's more there was something anti-intellectual about the letters and phone calls I received when I published articles about cancer care, recommending an assortment of remedies from Laetrile to meditation for stress. There was something unsettling about those shrill voices accusing the "cancer establishment," usually meaning the National Cancer Institute, the American Cancer Society, and/or Memorial Sloan-Kettering Cancer Center, of holding back on this or that "therapy" because its success might hurt business. I remember telling one, "Listen, I've been critical of the doctors and their teams too. But I've never met a doctor who wanted to kill me, and I've met a great many who wanted to cure me."

Norman Cousins might laugh himself loose from a rare degenerative disease called anky-losing spondylitis. But there was something impractical, even judgmental, about the idea that I could affect the course of a chronic illness, so prevalent and so feared that its very onset caused a modern woman (who was really not all that ill) to plan suicide on a Public TV documentary. This is what Holism tells us. It contends that, not only can psyche affect soma, and vice versa, but that we human beings are psychobiological unities, integrated within ourselves and our environments. Illness is an alien invasion of the positive harmony between mind and body; treatment is an effort to restore this harmony. Since mind and body work as one, there can be both an internal cause and cure, if only *you* take responsibility for finding them. The patient must minister to himself, not only for mind disease, ulcers, and a sore throat, but for heart disease ("Beware, stressy type A")—and now, for cancer.

All this made me envy my sister Ellen who reported in the 1960s that the only advantage of having cancer was that no one dared tell her *that* illness was psychosomatic. She got the kind of scornless treatment, the sympathetic care a real disease deserved.

The doctors had stopped giving me Adriamycin, the powerful "red devil" that had helped me so dramatically, but which can prove cardiotoxic. (No use to go to all that trouble not to die of cancer, only to die of heart failure.)

Bone scans and blood "markers," the medical indicators, showed my illness to be stable. But the more I missed the chemotherapy that had saved my life and worried lest the new, milder one would fail, the more my bones and muscles ached. I tried sitting in a swirling hot tub. I tried positive thinking, even a prayer or two.

Then my solemn, Harvard and National Cancer Institute-trained oncologist, Phil Cohen, suggested I make an appointment at Lynn Brallier's Stress Management Center, and I agreed. Lynn, a psychiatric nurse who had practiced biofeedback at the Psychiatric Institute of Washington, measured my bodily responses to stress (how much I sweated and my temperature changed, for instance, when I had to count backward from 300 by 17s) on tricky little biofeedback machines strapped to my hands, wrists, and head.

Somewhat to my surprise, the relaxation tapes she gave me to use two to six times a day turned out to be a smashing success. Hard-driving I, who sometimes did not even want to stop for lunch, found myself listening to them twice, even three times a day. As I heard that calm, low voice instructing me how to relax my muscles, from the tiny ones on my scalp, down to those in every toe, tension ebbed. At night, when I turned on another Brallier tape, "Suggestions for Restful Sleep" ("Say to yourself, I am at peace. I am at peace. You are falling asleep now, you are falling asleep"), I fell asleep.

When Lynn sent me to an adjoining office, skillful massage therapist Joan Delaney seemed to understand just how the various parts of my creaking body fit together. After she had manipulated the right muscles and pressed the right joints, I felt energized instead of tired. And when Lynn discussed my difficulties with me, or talked (unlike a traditional psychotherapist) to my doctor or my husband about them, she helped me stay on an even keel. She seemed to emphasize wellness, instead of illness, not what was bad with me, but what was good. I was even able to treat a third operation as though it were another bump on a bumpy road.

Intrigued, I began to look around a bit further. This was a world where herbal teas sit on coffee tables, acupuncture charts adorn walls. First names—there are few last names in the Land of Holism. Young people, mellifluous voices on tapes . . . tapes . . . and more tapes. An upbeat atmosphere of touching, yes even of love. A portion of professionalism, some solid training, and some solid help, especially for the often depressing day-to-day problems with family, friends, work, or just feeling punk, which beset the vulnerable, long-term patient. And most reassuring, a sometimes-held view that the help offered did not have to be an "alternative" to the conventional treatment that had helped, if not cured me. If I picked my helper carefully, I did not have to choose between the two.

In a Guided Imagery Workshop at the Washington School of Psychiatry, I tried to follow white-haired charismatic Marielle Fuller of the UCLA faculty when she suggested we form different pictures in our minds and then interpret what we saw, much like psychoanalytic patients analyzing dreams. With the rest of the group I did as she proposed, imagining myself on a large, sunny meadow, smelling the pungent cornflowers and sweet grass. I met a guide (a wizard). I dug in the ground and found an object. What was the object? Who—oh who—did I choose to give it to at this point in my life?

In my old khaki pants, I lay on the carpet in an empty living

67

room of a big house off Sixteenth Street, pushing various limbs against the floor, and trying to increase my ability to handle my body comfortably. Roger and Allison, the two young teachers, like their mentor, Israeli Moshe Feldenkrais, promise not a cure, but a new ability to use your entire muscular apparatus, and, as a result, more awareness of your movements and so lighter and freer patterns of movement. I followed the easy movements they suggested without trouble and was willing to try moving with more grace and balance, and thus to improve my health and well-being ("When a person is healthy, it turns out that he is not ill," says Feldenkrais). But they lost me completely during an interview in their kitchen after the class. Over herbal tea, they scoffed at scientific studies being done by "$40,000 a year researchers." They could not manage, they said, as I squirmed uncomfortably, in the "entrenched experimental paradigm." They preferred one based on "subjective experience."

In a simple Bethesda church I listened as former atomic scientist Jim Goure talked about "effective prayer." I gathered that this involved healing yourselves through finding the LIGHT, and healing others through visualizing the LIGHT in a neighbor. But the flowery spiritualist language and rapt approach were not for me ("I release all of my past, negatives, human relationships, fears, inner self, future and death in the LIGHT . . . I am a LIGHT being"). I left, unaffected by the experience.

The St. Francis Center Conference where I met jogger Harry seemed less way out, more in line with modern scientific attitudes. I could not accept all of controversial psychologist Lawrence LeShan's profile of a typical cancer patient: Someone who lacked closeness to one or both parents. Someone who has suffered a loss. Someone who feels hopeless, helpless, caught in the web of life who says: "If the egg drops on the rock—poor egg. If the rock drops on the egg—poor egg." *She is the egg.* I, and others I knew, had not acted absolutely like that woman. But parts of us might resemble her.

I read, I talked to experts. Whatever I did, and whatever I asked, my questions about the validity of applying holistic concepts to cancer kept coming back to the work being done by Carl and Stephanie Matthews-Simonton, then at the Cancer Counseling and Research Center at Fort Worth, Texas.

The Simontons have split now; she has taken the Cancer Counseling Center to Dallas, and he has moved to Los Angeles, where he works part time (and is heavily into skin diving). But even apart, the two remain the gurus of the cancer-holism connection. Other holistic therapists working with cancer patients quote them, discuss them, some emulate them. They have trained some 500 therapists, though they assume little responsibility for their trainees' work.

Psychologist Turner gave me a copy of their tape, on which I heard Carl Simonton inviting me to picture my strong, white cells eating up the weak, confused cancer cells. (I had never thought of cancer cells as weak and confused before.) Fellow patients in clinic waiting rooms or hospital corridors repeatedly asked if I had tried the Simonton techniques—they had, they would say, and they found them helpful. One cancer counselor, Dr. Wendy Schain, has reported that two out of five cancer patients mention the Simontons' therapy, and I believe it. When I interviewed Dr. Bernard Fox, the éminence grise who manages the National Cancer Institute's social science field studies and statistics program, he refused to lump together the sort of self-help therapies I inquired about vis-à-vis cancer and call them "holistic," as he felt that term is too poorly defined. Instead, this psychologist and epidemiologist, the author of the most highly regarded survey of psychological factors and cancer incidence, referred to "Simonton-type approaches."

Luckily for me, the Simontons were scheduled to come to Washington. I say luckily, for I would have found it difficult to travel to Texas to interview them and observe their treatment. And I would have found it expensive to participate ($1,900 for a ten-day course, and that would not include hotel costs for myself and spouse, who would have to come too).

In the course of an interview with Dr. Carl Simonton at a colleague's suburban home, his guest appearance on a radio talk show, and a packed day-long seminar at the University of

69

Maryland sponsored by an organization called Quest, I got the chance to see the Simontons in action, hear them out, and see them interact with their public.

He is a fortyish physician trained as a radiation oncologist, with brown curly hair and beard, wire-rimmed glasses, a penchant for four-letter expletives, and a willingness to appear on a platform in his jogging shorts. A Southern Baptist preacher's son, he has given up practicing radiation oncology; now he describes himself as someone who works with cancer patients using lifestyle counseling. She is a hard-driving, brainy, articulate young brunette in a California-smart white suit; though she is in a doctoral program, she has yet to receive her Ph.D. in clinical psychology.

At their research center, they are conducting what he emphasizes is a pilot study, which grew out of work begun when he was a resident at the University of Oregon more than ten years ago. There he noticed that some patients lacked hope; they did not seem to want to get well. The Simontons tried a new method to motivate a sixty-one-year-old man with advanced throat cancer who was taking radiation therapy.

The man was very weak, his weight had dropped from 130 to 98 pounds, he could barely swallow. Carl outlined a program of relaxation and mental imagery for him (similar to those his wife had found were used to motivate people in business). He was to set aside three blocks of time each day, first to compose himself by sitting quietly and telling each muscle group to relax, head to foot. Then in this more relaxed state, he was to picture himself in a pleasant, quiet place from nature, by a creek or waterfall, on a beach. Next, he was to picture his cancer vividly, and then his treatment—millions of tiny bullets of energy hitting his cells, including his weaker, more confused cancer cells. Last, and most important, he was to picture his body's white blood cells coming in, swarming over the cancer cells, picking up the dead and dying ones, and flushing them out of his body through his liver and kidneys. He was to visualize his cancer decreasing in size and his health returning.

The patient, who continued radiation therapy, responded

dramatically; he gained weight and his cancer progressively disappeared. The relaxation-imagery technique the Simontons used with him is still the centerpiece of their approach. It is combined with other activities and treatments designed to teach people to live in more healthy ways—exercise, diet, regular (usually group) counseling sessions, and a goodly dose of play. Patients learn to use such tools "smart" instead of "dumb." Too much exercise, for instance, can make you feel worse, the right amount can make you feel better. Overall, they are encouraged to probe and examine their lives, identifying what behaviors they might change to live fuller and more healthy lives, and seeing what "secondary benefits," like loving concern or needed rest, they get from their illness, and how they might substitute other ways than illness to meet their needs.

Gentleness is the key, "Be gentle with yourself," says Carl. "You did not get sick overnight, and you cannot get well overnight." Patients must continue under the care of a primary oncologist. The goals are 1) to alter the course of the patients' disease; 2) to improve their quality of life; 3) to improve their quality of death. Patients, some of whom remain in treatment with them for several years, are not pushed to a point where they feel uncomfortable; the idea is to support and care for them while they participate in their own treatment and change at their own pace.

All this is based on the theory held by the Simontons and others, that cancer is not a disease that strikes out of the blue. It develops, they hold, out of a complex interaction between our personality traits and the stressful life events we encounter. Our immune systems, nature's first line of defense, form the link between the two. During the course of a lifetime, cancer cells develop in all of us; usually they are surrounded and conquered by the cells of our immune system. If we are stressed by a demanding boss or a nagging spouse, our central nervous system can suppress this immune system. Hormonal balances can further suppress them.

This happens most often, according to the Simontons, to people with so-called "cancer-prone personalities." Like Law-

71

rence LeShan, whom I had heard a few weeks before, and physicians who since the second century A.D. have connected cancer with melancholia or black bile, they describe these people as those with poor self-images, who bottle up their resentments, have trouble forgiving and forming long-term relationships, and most important, have lost a serious love object or life role six to eighteen months before their diagnosis. (All of the forty new patients who come to the Simonton Center each year must fill out a form identifying the major life events of this period.) As a result they feel hopeless and helpless. In a sense their despair is turned inward toward their body cells. These cells become vulnerable to stress, and to cancer.

The Simontons say their pilot study results across the board thus far show their patients, all of whom suffered advanced malignancies, live twice as long as those reported currently in the literature (or "historical controls"). Carl Simonton told a recent Australian medical meeting that 71 of his breast cancer patients lived an average of 38.5 months as opposed to the same 19 months lived by historical controls. But the NCI's Bernard Fox pointed out that Simonton patients are those who are well enough and can afford to travel to their Texas center and sit through a program; yet they compare these patients not with a specific set of controls—that's hard to do—but with all patients, including those on their deathbeds. What's more, only a fraction of the men and women invited into the program accept. Possibly they feel less depressed and are indeed more well than those who fear, as Fox put it, they "could not take ten days of that stuff."

The Simontons contend their patients do more than live longer. They also live a more vibrant, better quality of life, and die in a better, less painful way. Stephanie told of a patient who worked all day, came home, and died peacefully that night. Carl stressed the importance of their "quality" approach, comparing it to that of many oncologists in major medical centers dependent on study funds who must keep patients on this combination of drugs or that according to the study protocol, until they die,

72

regardless of the quality of their lives. Bernard Fox simply says he has yet to see any Simonton quality of life study results; their reports, he notes, are anecdotal.

One thing is clear: the Simontons are not your usual medical team. They are a happening. They lead a movement. Their audiences seem rapt, adoring, uncritical ("I am Dorothy, 37, and I really called to thank you, sir, for your book. It showed me I am responsible for not letting cancer into my body"). When Stephanie Simonton told some 500 people, the majority of them cancer patients and counselors, at College Park that she hoped a cure for cancer would *not* be found, as a cure for polio had been, I was shocked, and so was a friend, a fellow patient. But most of the audience seemed to accept her, to my mind, cruel reasoning that such a vaccine-like cure for our sufferings would mask the societal issues involved, such as the stressful ways we bring up children, or the manner in which we allocate medical funds. One woman responded, "Thank you Stephanie, for your excellent presentation and for your guts."

The personal changes they have made in their lives mirror their teachings. He must, says Carl Simonton, focus on what is important to him as patients must focus on what is important to them. Maintaining his health must be his own first priority; the best teaching is done through role modeling, and if he destroys his own health (by living in a questionable marriage) he will be a terrible teacher. Now, "I put my own health up against that of any thirty-eight-year-old oncologist."

Like most causists, the Simontons are defensive about some of the criticisms a skeptical medical community has leveled against them. "The handwriting is on the wall," Carl Simonton explains, "we need to do research in new areas." No one has ever attempted before to alter the course of malignancy through psychological and lifestyle therapy, and people want answers from him in just ten year's time! "We're trying to find them. We don't have answers. No. We have questions. Jesus Christ, this is a brand new area!" He has been responsible; he has kept his nose pretty clean over the years. He does not, he reports, appreciate the "pot shots" people at major institutions level at him; he finds them annoying. It would be more helpful for the powers that be

73

to fund more behavioral studies. He does not, for example, know of one study on the effect of exercise on cancer. He thinks the National Cancer Institute must be spending a tiny percentage of its billion dollar budget on behavioral studies, perhaps 1 percent (an NCI spokesperson estimated it is spending somewhat less than 1 percent, which is less than $10 million).

The layman-reader, especially the seriously ill cancer patient desperate for clues, can be baffled by reports of studies attempting to link psychological factors, such as stress, and cancer. Common sense tells me that many people I know who are not depressed at all, including innocent children, develop ugly cancers; conversely many depressed, seemingly helpless, hopeless people go about their business, cancer-free. Common sense tells me I do not fit into Stephanie Simonton's description of the breast cancer patient: A "nice" person who does not express her sadness and vulnerability (here I am writing about it all) and is confused about her role in life. Common sense tells me that my perky, barking Corgi dog Patrick died sadly and suddenly of lung cancer last winter, and he did not even smoke, much less suffer depression.

Riffling through the voluminous literature, my doubts were heightened by studies like Robert J. Keehn's, which found the great stress of captivity suffered by prisoners of war did *not* accelerate malignancies and other degenerative changes in later years. Still, my bone pains *do* increase when I am tensely trying to perform my best on a television show. And they *do* ebb after I laugh my way through as funny a movie as *King of Hearts*.

Carl Simonton bases his work on an amalgam from the scientific literature. Generally, he cites the pioneering studies of Hans Selye, which describe the way the body is alarmed by stress, resists it, and finally when the stress is severe enough, looses its ability to resist; the life chart developed by Thomas H. Holmes linking life change events like the death of a spouse to illness—the more serious the event, the more serious the illness; and the widely known Meyer Friedman–Ray Rosenmann conclusion that "type A" strivers who live their life by the calendar

74

and clock and do everything rapidly are prime candidates for heart disease.

More specifically, he praises LeShan's profile of the anxious cancer patient who cannot express hostility and has arrived at a "no exit" place. He also relies on C.B. Thomas' work at Johns Hopkins linking a lack of closeness to parents with tumor development; on A.H. Schmale's results predicting that women with helplessness-prone personalities would develop cancer of the cervix; E.M. Blumberg's findings that patients with fast-growing tumors were characteristically more defensive and tense than patients with slow-growing tumors; and D.M. Kissen's research tying a poor ability to discharge emotions to lung cancer. So many animal studies have shown that electric shock and other stresses increase tumor growth, Simonton holds, that no more need be done.

Not so, say the UCLA School of Medicine's Department of Psychiatry's Drs. David Wellisch and Joel Yager in *Controversies in Cancer Treatment* (edited by UCLA oncologist Dr. Michael Van Skoy-Mosher, published by G.K. Hall). They ask, "Is there a cancer prone personality?" and answer, "No." Available evidence does not support the concept of such a creature; it is at best inconclusive. They hold that thus far no one study has been sufficiently well designed to remove the substantial doubts as to which personality factors might lead to cancer for what specific reason, or precisely how "black boxes" like the immune or hormonal system work to link these factors, personality and stress, to cancer. The best psychodynamicists have been able to do thus far is offer interpretations as to why people who have already developed cancer have done so, but not why they, rather than others, have developed the disease.

The UCLA team explains the mind-baffling issues that bedevil psychological cancer research. Many methodological problems increase the complexities: Not all cancers are the same, indeed, different tumors can be found in one organ (I have suffered two types of primary breast cancer); yet many important studies have treated diverse cancers equally. What's more, although epidemiological factors, like age, smoking, exposure to industrial toxins, or social class, have been associated with different cancers, they have rarely been controlled (or systematically compared) in studies of the cancer-prone personality. They may affect performance on the psychological tests researchers use, usually tests conveniently available, but not meaningful perhaps, for use with cancer patients.

Studies of animals, where conditions are far more controllable than in human beings, are often contradictory (some show stress improves resistance to cancer in animals, others that it reduces that resistance). Retrospective studies are all suspect; the knowledge that you *have* cancer can profoundly color a patient's emotional state, and the cancers themselves can cause psychological changes; depression may be a consequence rather than a cause. Even the findings of a very careful researcher like David Kissen who tried to interview patients before they were told of their disease, have not been supported by others.

The studies that merit most careful consideration are the few prospective ones, predicting who will fall victim to cancer. Dr. Caroline Thomas' work at Johns Hopkins linking a lack of closeness to parents to the development of cancer in a group of 913 white male physicians, is probably, according to UCLA's Wellisch and Yager, the most important. Yet it suffers many shortcomings in the lack of reported controls for potential cancer causes like smoking or a family history of cancer.

Finally, the role of immunological and hormonal causation in cancer is very obscure and complex, more a statement of faith than fact. The immune system is composed of a great variety of cells and hormones, there are two types of T-cell lymphocytes, for instance, and when one is suppressed it may augment activity in another part of the immune system. The most important, prevalent cancers have not been found to be more frequent in people with immunological disorders.

The psychologist who heads the National Cancer Institute's Behavioral Medicine Branch, Dr. Sandra Levy, agrees. There is a clear link, she says, between higher cortical functions and biological response, but it is very complex, and scientists do not yet fully understand it. The Simontons and others like them are making a "quantum leap" in practicing therapies assuming a direction of influence from mind to body—that imagining your cure can actually bring it about.

Dr. Levy's branch spends some $4 million a year on behavioral cancer research, including a wide variety of problems like teenage smoking or the control of pain in terminal care; there is additional behavioral research going on as part of other studies in this huge government institute. Her immediate boss, Dr. William Terry, points out that the NCI is focusing on those aspects of human behavior and lifestyle that now account for 30 percent of cancer deaths—habits such as cigarette smoking and the excessive ingestion of alcohol.

Sandra Levy herself is interested in biological mediators between behavior and disease, like cancer; she with the NCI's breast cancer chief, Dr. Marc Lippman, has begun to study the connection between emotional response of breast cancer patients to their disease and the length of their survival. However, like Sloan-Kettering's Dr. Jimmie Holland, she feels that no replicated findings have related altered emotional state to cancer in humans. Admitting to the rise of a self-help zeitgeist in the land and the popularity of Simonton-type methods, she feels there may be a need in the field for a well-designed, controlled, clinical trial done by dispassionate, professional researchers. Medical scientific standards of quantification and replicability must be met, as they were met in the Laetrile trials.

Until this is done, what about us, the cancer patients, hanging in there? The naturalistic approach of increasing our bodies' own fight against disease appeals to us. The awful thing about cancer is that it is so sly and nasty, creeping crazily around inside of us. If we can outwit it through our own hope, our own conviction, our own imagination, we will gain back the sense of self-control so important to us.

Some experts say that even if the Simonton-type methods do not cure cancer, patients who try them often emerge revitalized, renewed in spirit. Perhaps people simply are helped by a switch from the often cold, scary ambience of high medicine to one of warmth and caring. (A patient I know was devastated when her oncologist seemingly failed to recognize her in the clinic elevator.)

Besides, their argument runs, the Simonton-type treatments are so attractive because, unlike toxic chemotherapy, for example, they offer something for nothing (except money). If they give you hope and cannot harm you, why not try them? Other experts answer that they *can* harm you. Patients have been known to abandon conventional treatment to try them, only to collapse. Sloan-Kettering's Dr. Holland adds there can be more subtle harm done. Patients who already may feel severely punished can be made to feel guilty if they think their cancer is their own fault. They can feel guiltier still if their cancer progresses despite their self-help efforts. This guilt is scarcely alleviated by the group leaders nurse-consultant Marie Manthey told me about. These doctors and their coworkers accuse patients with unremitting pain of choosing to fail at imagery because "they want to be in pain." Ms. Manthey fears they do this because they want to shuffle their own inability to deal with failure to cure onto their patients.

Carl Simonton himself is well aware of the guilt issue. He says guilt permeates our society, parents, teachers, peers, even perhaps our religions can make us feel guilty about this or that. What he tells his patients is that just as in the birth canal they participated, albeit unconsciously, in their own births, so they participated, albeit unconsciously, in the growth of their cancers, and can participate in the process of regaining their health. They must recognize their human limits in understanding the unconscious quality of all this; they must learn to trust that just as they were born, their health can be reborn; they must learn to trust, as Einstein put it, that "the universe is kind." But who knows what effect all those other Simonton-type therapists out there are having on patients?

What I have concluded after several months of investigation, is that some parts of the holistic explosion have something to offer me and my fellow cancer patients. At the very least, they can be palliative, helping us relax and deal better with our difficulties, in sum, increasing our sense of wellness instead of illness. At the most, they could help improve our health, though we must wait for more solid proof before we raise our hopes too high. Meanwhile, we can tap into them not as alternatives, but as adjuncts to our treatment.

Caveat emptor, friend patient, once again. Be as painstaking in checking the credentials of those who offer you holistic services as you would be of other practioners, whether as leader of a group or as individual therapist. Be sure you are comfortable with their assumptions, both medical and spiritual. Be wary of therapists and others parroting them who make you weep because you cannot get your act together. Who is to judge if your cancer is your "fault" or a phenomenon of nature? After a second cancerous obstruction was diagnosed, a woman I met sat on the john all day crying as she read articles in popular magazines about people who had gotten the upper hand over their cancers. Why couldn't *she* do that?

Be wary, too, of therapists who would deprive you of what modern medicine has to offer you, who will not work with doctors. If therapists are true holists, they will acknowledge the strong powers of the body as well as of the mind and the uncertainties of the complex relation between the two. As astute California oncologist Dr. Michael Van Skoy-Mosher puts it, "What goes on below the neck is just as important as what goes on above it. The function of the neck is to connect the two."

CHAPTER 6

"SIGNIFICANT OTHERS": A PART OF THE MAIN

No one knows better than the hanging-in patient that no man or woman is an island, entire of itself. No one knows better than the patient whose life depends on extended, esoteric, at times debilitating treatment, that each of us is a piece of the continent, a part of the main. The bell signaling involvement in mankind tolls for the hanging-in patient with singular force and intensity.

This is because we become more keenly aware of the way lives intertwine as every month and every year passes. The French have a saying that translates "to say goodbye is to die a little." We hope our deaths will diminish those who outlive us, at least a little. Meanwhile, our continued involvement with groups we value—our families, close friends, any of the human beings the therapists have antiseptically dubbed "significant others"—increases our ability to handle serious illness and its consequences.

If we continue to be involved with people we care about, if they ask us to do things with and for them, we know that though

81

we may have to change the way of life we lived before we became sick, we do not have to retire from that life. We can lead, as the public television show I participated in was titled, "A Different Kind of Life," limited by illness, but not ill, closer to death than many others, but alive and kicking.

Appearing on this TV program, my husband Jerry explained what this different life with me is like. He reported that as we leave the beach cottage we love on the Delaware shore each Labor Day weekend, I now muse, "I wonder if I'll ever see the beach house again." I did not used to wonder that. He added that, living with me, he sometimes feels like the ground crew for a supersonic plane: When I'm off and flying I'm going at top speed, but when I land (often flat on my bed upstairs at 5:00 P.M.), I need a certain amount of service between flights. My energy is limited, and he needs to do many things that I used to do (like washing the dinner dishes), so I will have the strength to do what I want.

I think that what he was saying was that in the "different life," you are invariably dependent on other people. For virtually all of us hanging-in patients, total independence is impossible. Our macho culture's emphasis on independence might make this seem bad, but it is not. On the contrary, some dependency, a positive dependency that recognizes the limits illness places on you and the help you need, may be a sign of maturity, of a pragmatic willingness to accept your situation.

What would not be good for you would be to refuse to lead this "different" life with others, to prefer, for whatever reason to remain "sick." It used to be that illness was temporary. You fell sick, you either got well or died in short order, and during that time, you gave up behaving as a responsible adult. Now that you hang in for long periods, it's a new ball game, a ball game in which illness can have its own "secondary gains." Refusing to make the switch from living as a "sick" person, to living as a "different" one, may satisfy some of these "secondary" unconscious needs—to behave as a child, stay home from a dull job, curl up in bed, be the center of attention and get taken care of. It does not permit us maximum independence and freedom of choice. It does not permit us to resume our adult responsibilities.

Family! The most significant of the others in our lives are usually found in this embattled entity. With divorce rates rising, and men and women experimenting with all kinds of novel living arrangements, the family as an institution seems to have fallen from grace.

No matter. We hanging-in patients usually look to our families for refuge and support, however we define them. The world may be, as the poet put it, a "darkling plain, swept with confused alarm of struggle and flight, where ignorant armies clash by night," but at home we hope to find a measure of certitude and peace, as well as help for pain.

I think this is even truer for cancer patients than for other long-term patients. For the armies out there are still, alas, more ignorant about cancer than other diseases. As we shall see further in the next chapter, people fear and dread cancer. Mythicizing the disease, they feel vulnerable to it. Asked for their first thought when the word "cancer" was mentioned, a group of university medical and nursing students, who after all, had seen a good deal of many terrible afflictions, answered: pain, death, hopelessness, dependency, loneliness.

If you want to know what's really happening in the world, read the "Advice to the Lovelorn" columns. In 1980, a forty-year-old Californian wrote *Dear Abby* after reading a letter from a woman who hesitated to buy a home in which the previous owner had died of cancer because she feared she might "catch" the disease. Similarly, she recalled that after her hysterectomy ten years earlier her friends had sent notes, cards, and flowers, but very few came to see her. Her first day out of the house, she was slowly walking to the end of the block when she saw one of her neighbors grab her little girl and hurry her home. Safely through the screen door she shouted, "How are you?" "I'm just fine, thank you." "Does your doctor think it has any-

83

thing to do with your smoking?" "No, I have always smoked with my mouth!"

Good for her; she kept her sense of humor. In the face of such ludicrous goings on, you cannot always do that. It is easy to see why many cancer patients feel safer, more protected within the inner circle of their families. As one young wife and mother told family therapist Dr. Robert Cantor (reported in his interesting book, *And A Time To Live*), "I feel surrounded by monsters of disease and despair. Ralph and those who love me are like an inner circle; they form a protective band around me. Without them, I'd be dead."

I know how she felt. I'm lucky enough never to have had someone drag a child away from me. My friends, even acquaintances on my block, are more sophisticated, more knowledgeable about cancer. But I cannot vouch for all of them, and I cannot vouch for whomever I might bump into tomorrow. Like most cancer patients, and it must be true of many other hanging-in patients as well, particularly those with obvious, "distasteful" disabilities, I feel safest in my nest.

"Mother, I am sorry to hear that you have been having pains lately," wrote my professor son Jon from Atlanta during my last pain-waxing period. "I hope you are feeling better now. It must be discouraging to have relapses. I am praying for your health. Now that I know Hebrew, I expect to be getting better results."

Darned if that letter, along with some weeks of rest, did not do the trick; I began to feel better. Even though my nest is an empty one, my two sons remain an integral part of my protective inner circle. I know they love me and stand ready to do what they can for me, but it helps when they let me know they are rooting for me.

More and more, cancer is regarded as a family affair. But problems arise when the family cannot always serve as a first line of defense. The disease hits family members individually and also as a unit, as must other diseases with unfortunate implications of disaster and death. It can strain these family members and attack the family's integrity as a working system.

Homeostasis is a word scientists use to describe the process whereby the human body tries to maintain a steady state in the face of environmental change, such as a change in temperature. If you jog in the sun and get too hot and uncomfortable, your skin senses this and sends a message to your brain. You perspire, getting rid of heat. You also probably stop jogging and move into the shade to rest. In the same way, a family senses change and tries in conscious and unconscious ways to maintain its internal balance.

Patients and families interact in this process in different ways. Like many other counselors, Grace Christ, Sloan-Kettering's chief social worker, feels that in dealing with cancer patients and their families, she sees people at their best. Again and again she is struck with the courage and nobility of these families, with their extraordinary empathy and support for each other.

I have seen such hanging-in families too. After a swim, I met Pat McEvoy in the health club dressing room adjusting her blond wig. When I ventured a comment about my short hair, which had grown back even though I was still on chemotherapy, she responded vigorously and cheerfully, telling me about herself, her mastectomy, and her busy family.

Pat, a lawyer and mother of five, remarried some months before her surgery. Her husband and her kids, who range in age from twelve to twenty, are doing splendidly. There have been a few changes; the younger children, she has noticed, touch her more than they used to, making sure she's there. She has taught her teenaged daughter to examine her own breasts. And all are perhaps a bit more solicitous. Her twenty-year-old son calls from Boston to play her guitar music he has recorded.

By and large, however, each member of the family continues cheerfully and coolly to do his own thing. Pat thinks this is because she's been open, but not scary about her illness, and because they are used to behaving independently, pitching in and taking care of each other, "It's the way I've raised them." She appreciates their good humor and their not allowing her to get depressed, "They joke with me. They ask, 'Mom, how are

85

you and your false boob?' Or they tell me that with my bald head I look like something out of *Star Wars*."

Not allowing depression seems to be a family characteristic much appreciated by us hanging-in patients. According to Harley Dirks, whom I knew as a widely respected Capitol Hill health staffer, his wife Ruthie is his partner in sickness and health. Through colostomy surgery, radiation, and chemotherapy, "she not only loves me and understands me but gets tough with me when I get depressed."

Families can get shocked into adjusting to the hanging-in subculture. A social worker remembers a young mother who, in prechemotherapy days, had a pelvic exoneration (which means, as my mother used to say, "everything out," including ovaries, uterus, and part of the intestine). She went home to West Virginia very depressed; she simply could not cheer up. Most of the day and a good bit of the night, she wept. When her two sisters came to see her, they wept too. One afternoon, they were sitting, crying, in the kitchen when her eight-year-old son came home from school and started to cry with them. Shocked, they pulled themselves together and stopped crying. So well did this young woman do subsequently, so trim and snappy did she look, that the hospital staff asked her to talk to their newer cancer patients about her experiences.

Yet it's true that families can be permanently hurt, even fragmented, by serious illness. They may organize themselves around the illness in a way that can lead to difficulty. One divorced friend of mine, for example, sensed that she was leaning too much on one of her older sons in inappropriate ways (asking him to rub her back, for instance). She switched gears and found other people to care for her before harm was done. At times, families cannot withstand the strain and breakup. After hearing one horror story about a husband who vanished after his wife's mastectomy, I reacted strongly, "She's better off without him!" But the bearer of the tale, a friend of the mastectomee, had a different view, "It's a bullshit society!"

That may be. I think that generally families with somewhat less than average strengths and abilities may not fare too well under stress, although they had managed adequately before. This was one message of a poignant booklet, *Listen to the Children!*, by a New York service organization called Cancer Care. Reporting on a study of the impact on the mental health of 88 children under the age of nineteen of a parent's catastrophic illness, in this case, well-advanced cancer, the group found that such illness can overwhelm some parents, even with adequate parenting skills, making them anxious about what to tell the children about death and angry at their lot. Others react with calm strength and insight, sharing the ramifications of illness, being quick to recognize and respond to danger signs.

For those with barely average strength and ability to parent, the incapacitation of either a mother or father often fragments whatever the two had managed together. All they can do now is cope with the illness; children can become secondary, ignored, resented. For those immature, perhaps disturbed parents who even in good times manage only a delicate balance, the incapacitation can destroy the tenuous security they have built for their children.

When these things are true, children can send out a variety of warning signals. Sixteen-year-old Thomas's school grades decline; he becomes extremely tense, fearful, often angry. Fearful, immature Roger, eleven years old, develops pain resembling that suffered by his mother. Twelve-year-old Mary eats voraciously; by gaining weight, she tries to force her mother's attention from her father's sickroom. Eleven-year-old Kirk begins to steal money from his home and from his neighbors. Nine-year-old Tom has behaved like a sad old man since his mother returned, visibly weakened, from the hospital.

The longer the illness, the worse the effect. There was a significant correlation between the length of the illness and the children's behavior difficulties. Although those six- to ten-year-olds who were kept *unaware* of the nature of their parent's illness had more behavior problems, so did the older children of eleven to nineteen years of age who *were* aware. "Awareness," in this study, meant the child had been told the diagnosis and had also been told that the parent was going to die, a real "sock it to 'em" message. Clearly, what all the children were told was less crucial than how they were informed and then involved in family matters.

The researchers felt that adolescents differed from younger children in their reaction to the message because their growing pains were compounded as they were buffeted by parental illness just at a stage in their lives when increasing self-responsibility and independence are being tentatively established. This may be. To me the difference says that we are all human, children and adults. As the analytic literature points out, little children often perceive death as transitory, related to sleep or rest. Not fully grasping the cruel message, the younger children did better when they were simply told, and made to feel included, rather than pushed aside during whispered grown-up conversations. Understanding the message, the adolescents, like adults, were upset and fearful that their world might come crashing down about them. Both little children and adolescents, like adults, gained hope and were able to behave more maturely when the message was more tactfully, more gently presented. Indeed they might—they could—survive.

So families, like individuals, are different. Their first differences are obvious: families, like individuals, find themselves at different ages and stages of development when illness strikes.

Young people, just starting careers and families, find themselves behind a different eight ball than middle-aged folk who have established family "launching centers" (with their first or even last child gone). They have less financial and job security, they are not even used to being sick. Sadly, their paths are blocked just as they are starting out.

Middle-aged, "launching center" families have another set of problems. With their children gone, with their own parents becoming ill or dependent, perhaps demanding attention in nursing homes, they are trying to establish new interests, even new careers. Illness now drains their energy and keeps them from a fresh start. They suffer in a different way from the young family whose nine-year-old daughter develops a facial tic and nervous cough when her mother's breast cancer metastasizes. They suffer in a still different way from the physically aging family already trying to deal with failing eyesight and hearing, memory problems, and numerous joint and bone pains. New, chronic illness may simply be more than older families can handle.

If some differences between hanging-in patients are spread out for all to see, others are far more subtle. People do not, as we all know, suffer illness in a vacuum. They are what they are; they have been behaving in a certain way, sometimes for a very long while; illness only brings forth what was there before. Pat McEvoy raised her five children to take care of themselves and act in a self-reliant way, as she pointed out to me. She was on her own for a decade; the kids had already learned not to lean too heavily on her and to face small crises while she was at law school and at work. A strong family, they are learning easily to become part of the hanging-in subculture.

Family sociologists have outdone themselves, it seems to me, in trying to characterize families. They divide them into motor and cerebral groups, into open and closed systems, into mother- or father- or child-centered units. Surveying many such typologies, The University of Rochester's Lawrence Fisher does us the favor of combining them into different sorts of "family clusters." These are as follows: *constricted* types, with restricted emotional lives; *internalized* types, who focus inward and view the world with pessimism, hostility, and threat; *object-focused* types, who overemphasize or rely excessively on children, the outside community, or themselves; *impulsive* types, marked by a troublesome adolescent or young adult who displaces his anger on parents or community and acts out in a socially undesirable way; *childlike,* often young family types, needy and dependent, who never completely separate from their family of origin; and the rarer *chaotic* type, usually lower-class, unstable people, often jobless, with members coming in and out of the family unit.

Such classifications leave many, including me, a bit confused and sad. Of course, they emphasize maladaptive tendencies, since they derive largely from studies of people referred for some sort of mental health treatment. Dr. Susan Mellette's way of thinking about how cancer affects families appeals to me more. Even its downbeat aspects seem more upbeat; I find it less jargonistic, more in tune with Ogden Nash's classic, very human definition: "A family is a unit composed not only of children, but of men, women, an occasional animal, and the common cold."

To start with, this Medical College of Virginia oncologist affirms that most family members *are* able to marshall their resources to come to grips with the new problems of illness. She bases this good news on a family adjustment study done at her college. Comparing degrees of adjustment, research teams found that patients living at home with their immediate families have much higher and less variable ratings than patients who were shunted off to live with others. They enjoyed more support, exhibited less signs of stress and signs of crisis. They ranked higher on an emotional adjustment scale too.

Dr. Mellette describes families who *do* have difficulties realistically. There is the *Over Reactive Family*. Nothing is too much for them to do for the patient, no expense too great to bear. I saw one such family in the adjoining room when I was last in the hospital. That room was chock full of flowers and cards. So many people crowded into it at visiting hours, with such excited conversation, that I wondered how the patient would feel when she tried to get back to normal, or when—down the road when her family had, perhaps, exhausted its energy—she needed continuing attention and support.

Then there's the *Over Protective*, even the *Pseudo-Protective* family. I recognize this family too. Some of those closest to me, my husband especially, would overprotect me if I let them, drive for me, run errands for me. My good mother, who has spent a lifetime doing things for other people, would be in my house all the time if we lived in the same city (we don't), and she weren't having her own health problems. Dr. Mellette pointed out that sometimes overprotection is a sign, not only of good intentions, but of underlying pathology. Adult children, for example, may finally establish their own independence by making the parent the child. The *Masochistic Family* contains a member, usually a spouse, who wants to protect the patient at personal cost: the husband who gives up his lifework to take care of his wife; the wife who sits unnecessarily by her husband's hospital bed all day and night and won't even accept a cot from the nursing staff.

On the other hand, in the *Angry Family*, a member turns some of the grief and anger he or she naturally feels, against the patient (why did this have to happen to us?). A visiting nurse describes an elderly wife who kept chewing her husband out because he had smoked and so developed cancer, "I could just hit you for smoking all those years." Dr. Mellette tells of a woman with metastatic breast cancer whose husband actually beat her up, he was so angry at her disease. This story at least had a happy ending. The beating was never repeated, and he came to care for her later when such care was necessary with amazing skill and tenderness.

Finally, there's the family that denies the disease and becomes *Over Dependent* on the patient, expecting the usual or even the impossible of him or her. One such husband brought his lady friend to the hospital while he visited his wife, expecting them to be polite to each other.

At an American Cancer Society conference in Atlanta, I met a brainy blonde nurse called Barbara Giacquinta. Chairperson of Pace University's Nursing School Graduate Division, Barbara is a Ph.D. who took care of her own mother when she was hanging in with cancer. As a result of that and other experiences, she developed a model, a way of thinking about how a family facing serious disease behaves, the phases it goes through, and hurdles it must overcome.

She sent me a nursing journal article describing this model, which is well known in cancer care circles. I like it. It seems realistic, helpful to professionals, particularly since it is prefaced with a warning to nurses not to misuse it by stereotyping complex human behavior and distancing themselves from their patients. Since it is not overly jargony, and chronologically structured—though a family can go through several phases at a time—it is helpful to patients and their families, as well.

As it lives with cancer, says Barbara Giacquinta, the family must first face the *impact* of that disease. The shock and strain the bad news naturally brings can cause family members to act anxious or agitated, or to withdraw, sulking and guilty. A husband becomes an insomniac and soon needs sedation to sleep at night. An older son begins to drink or smoke too much pot, taking refuge in alcohol or drugs. A daughter suffers crying spells.

The entire group may become disorganized, or key members can come forward to help others. I know I depended a good deal on my brother who is a doctor (a psychoanalyst) in Baltimore. I depended on him to talk to my doctors for me. I depended on him to glean information, since, as I have pointed out, the doctors did not always talk to me as I wished—candidly, but tactfully and optimistically. (This was important at the time: Some families become angry, even resentful of doctors, blaming them for the news they convey or, recognizing that the doctor controls the patient's fate, they act overly polite and deferential and don't dare to ask even ordinary questions.) But as the years have gone on and I have gained confidence in my hanging-in status, I've not needed my brother to mediate for me. I've learned to give doctors strong cues as to what I want to know (see chapter 3).

Despair is the hurdle the family needs to overcome in this impact phase. Other people can help by fostering hope. Barbara Giacquinta says hope is composed both of the feeling that the family can live with the disease, and the sense of security that modern medicine, with its surgery, radiation, and drug therapies, may help. It's true; even if a patient or family is in shock, they are quick to perceive hope, which allows them to imagine a future in those around them. Conversely, they are quick to perceive hopelessness. They avoid pessimistic nurses and leave despairing doctors if they can.

Functional disruption may occur as the family adjusts to a different lifestyle. Household management may suffer, children's daily needs may not be met as a husband takes over the traditional wifely role. Or egos suffer as a wife becomes the family breadwinner, or attempts to overprotect her husband.

Isolation is the hurdle the family needs to overcome as it goes about the business of daily living, trying to stay stable and autonomous. If family members find it hard to talk to each other, if they go their separate ways, they are less able to reach out to support systems, like support groups in the community. Anything other people can do to foster family cohesion helps, whether it be helping a couple define their real needs and priorities, or finding the social and material resources they need. In Minneapolis, Minnesota, North Memorial Medical Center nurses Judi Johnson and Pat Norby run a highly successful program called "We Can Weekend" to help families overcome the isolation hurdle. Twice a year they take a group of about 25 families, each with at least one cancer patient, away on a weekend packed with lessons and projects about cancer facts and fallacies or relaxation and exercise techniques. Emphasizing communication between patient, family, and health team, "We Can Weekend" teaches families to express their feelings, to like themselves, to live with limits, to tap helping resources.

A *search for meaning,* the third phase of the Giacquinta model, could, it seems to me, take place at any time in the hanging-in process. This is the intellectualization of cancer, the attempt to gain intellectual mastery over the disease process.

A sister goes to the library to bone up on cancer. A husband consults so many specialists that he becomes confused and does not know what to do. A grandmother blames the patient for drinking too much alcohol or diet soda; again, that insidious "It's your fault!" As each family member becomes more involved with the patient, he is more vulnerable, more conscious of his own mortality. My son Jon says he became more aware of the limits of time when my cancer began seriously to metastasize. He broke up with the young woman he had been going with

93

for four years, "We weren't getting anywhere and I was *thirty!*"

Others can help families vault the vulnerability hurdle by supplying them with information they need, or leading them to it. For most people, this means more than giving them a bunch of pamphlets. My elder son, Jeremy, stopped worrying when a doctor defined his chances of getting breast cancer during a regular checkup. Harley Dirks reports that he and his family have received 109 pamphlets during treatment, and very little else. What they want is information that will enable them to put their trust in the treatment methods being used on him, "I want to be excited about my therapy, worked out with those who are involved in saving my life."

Informing others, the fourth phase, could take place any time in the hanging-in process, before the family has overcome the hurdles of despair, isolation, and vulnerability, or afterward. To me it encompasses the family's relations with friends and acquaintances.

If other people bombard family members with questions they cannot answer or pressure them with intrusive suggestions that they seek this or that medical opinion or alternative treatment, the family may retreat—another hurdle to overcome. For me, the best way to avoid retreat has been to speak out frankly about my illness, and to tell people exactly what I am doing to fight it, when they ask. Candor has been my ally; my family has followed suit. But some patients and their families need professional counseling help in sorting out their feelings about their illness. In this way, they gain the courage they need to deal with outside influences (see chapter 5).

In the fifth Giacquinta phase, *engaging emotions*, volatile feelings can come to the surface. As the illness changes family goals and satisfactions, as positions of security shift, families can worry about losing control. Displaying emotions, they may feel helpless, "Everything that can be done has been done." Helplessness is the fifth hurdle.

It's only when people suppress their feelings and lose touch with each other, that people run into real trouble. When they are helped in solving problems, when they can acknowledge and express their emotions, there is no loss of control. Former Senator Birch Bayh reports that his wife Marvella wrote and spoke and counseled women with breast cancer because she wanted them to know that they were not failures if they doubted, cried, or yelled at their husbands. She wanted them to know these were all very normal things.

She also wanted them to know that their husbands usually would not desert them if they lost a breast. Bayh believes that although this happens once in a while in a problem-ridden marriage, usually good marriages, wherein the partners are candid with each other and express their differences, are made better, "That was what happened in our case."

There is a tendency to romanticize the problems surrounding sex. But a hardnosed study of 31 couples conducted by a UCLA team and reported on in the *American Journal of Psychiatry* in 1978 generally bears out the Bayhs' approach. True, the response of husbands to their spouse's mastectomy can precipitate a crisis of profound proportions. Sexuality and intimacy can be put under severe stress and negatively altered; roughly half the men in the study thought, for instance, that mastectomy had reduced their wife's orgasmic potential.

Basically, the study results were encouraging. Most men, especially those who were least distant, most involved in decision making, or most frequent hospital visitors, or who had seen their wives nude since surgery (six of the thirty-one had not), coped well with the stresses mastectomy brought. Their relationships remained sound.

If the patient gets worse and either goes to the hospital or has to be taken care of at home, the family goes through two more phases: *reorganization,* in which the husband or wife or children take on new tasks; and *framing memories,* the attempt to remember the very ill person in healthier, happier times. Sometimes looking at pictures, leafing through scrapbooks, and storytelling help to crystallize the patient's relations over the years with those he cares about. Family members may need professional counseling as they try to cooperate and support each other and give the ill person a clear identity.

"We few, we happy few, we band of brothers." Shakespeare, who plumbed the human soul so deeply, understood that friends can become family, especially in the heat of battle. Nowadays, with families separated and parents and children moving about frequently, we come to depend more and more on our friends when we face a crisis. They become our brothers—and sisters, uncles, and aunts.

Like family they overreact to our illness. Like family they seek to overprotect us, or expect too much of us. They may not live in the same house with us, but they can be more emotionally engaged with us than those who do. "Friends can be better than family. Friends *want* to be there. Family is just there," says Gene Rosenfeld, whose wife Chris acted like a sister to my friend Diana Michaelis as she hung in there—dropping in each day, filling prescriptions, taking her to the Georgetown University Hospital clinic for tests.

We usually find out who our real friends are when we fall ill. As we hang in, learning to live a "different" life, the men are really sifted from the boys.

Our experiences differ. NBC producer Leonard Probst reported in *The New York Times* that friends were his best medicine in a recovery period. They came to visit every day—morning, some afternoons, and always at night. He and his wife had so many offers to bring dinner, they had to ask friends to accommodate themselves to a crowded social schedule. They were offered summer visits at houses in Martha's Vineyard and Sagaponack. They received invitations to stay at intriguing places from Siesta Key to the Laurentian Mountains in Canada.

Most people are not celebrities to be contested for. "Dear Ann Landers," Chris's Mom, the mother of a leukemia patient wrote in 1980, "When a member of the family becomes seriously ill, friends and relatives often stop calling. Perhaps they are afraid they will say the wrong thing, or they find sick people depressing. Whatever the reason, they are nowhere around." Chris's

96

Mom makes an eloquent plea to family and friends, "BE THERE for them, please. Pay a visit, make a phone call, send a letter ... the most precious gift you can give is yourself."

Another Ann Landers correspondent, "Freeport, Ill.," in the same year wrote her family and friends about a reality that may affect anyone as the years pass, "When you first found out about my illness you came by to see me. Your concern and caring gave us all a great deal of emotional support. But where are you now? ... As time goes by, I need you MORE—not less. I don't want your pity, just your friendship." And Linda Eckley, a plucky woman whose breast cancer has metastasized to her brain, told me, "I used to hate the telephone. Now I wish it would ring."

My experience is somewhere in-between. No one offered me a summer villa, even at the beginning of my illness. But most of my friends have rallied round and haven't deserted me as the years have gone on. I agree with Leonard Probst that a good set of friends bring you themselves, their lives, and their dinners, the everyday things. I've particularly appreciated Charley and Shirley Seib showing up consistently with their good casseroles and conversation.

I've appreciated the unusual gesture or gift too: the shopping expedition early on with Judy Turner, when she took me to buy my first prosthesis and turned a dismal chore into a lark. Judy has a flair for fun. She writes a skiing column, and asked me to ski with her one day about an hour from Washington. I could not do that anymore, but I still remember the warm glow I felt as I flew down the hill, "Just whistle a Cole Porter tune," Judy advised.

The other day I felt the same glow when my college classmates, Ann Horvitz and Peggy Randol dropped by (Peggy from Baltimore), or when my lawyer-friend Edith Fierst touched base and made a lunch date. Old friends, who show their love and generosity, are like precious stones when you are hanging-in. Tina Fredericks, whom I've known since high school called out of the blue last year from Long Island. "We're going to Haiti," she announced. I hesitated, then agreed. "What if I collapse?" "Then I'll push the wheelchair," she volunteered. We had a ball, and needed no wheelchair. In fact, I felt better in sunny, creative Haiti.

I've appreciated the new friends I've made in this period, most of them younger people interested in the same things as I. Fred Register, with whom I wrote speeches for Secretary Shirley Hufstedler during a good year at the Department of Education. Ricki Green, the talented producer of the "A Different Kind of Life" television show. Both keep in touch; Fred by phone from California and Ricki here in town. I told Ricki once I felt like the biblical sage Ecclesiastes who wrote that he hated all his labor "wherein I labored under the sun, seeing I must leave it unto the man that shall come after me. And who knoweth whether he will be a wise man or a fool?" She, I said, was my wise man.

The Scriptures know it all, "One who visits the sick takes one-sixth of the illness away." This is usually true, but not always. A friend may feel uncomfortable around sickness and someone she perceives as threatened by death. Our society has not prepared her too well to face death. It is a society in which we color our hair to hide the grey, lift our faces to stretch away the wrinkles, and separate ourselves from impending death by relegating our parents and grandparents to nursing homes. So your friend shies away from you even if she can get herself to visit you. She distances herself from you, perhaps criticizing something you did (like not divorcing or quitting work or mourning your parents). If she acts differently, she feels she has a better chance of fending off disease and death.

I've learned that such a friend is really "scared," like the teasing friends of the "Rainbow Kids" we met in chapter 1. But most of the few who behaved this way at the beginning of my illness have gotten used to my hanging in; we are back to normal. Only one I cared about moved out of my life; this made me feel dreadful. Conversely, some people are attracted to illness like moths to a flame. They are fascinated by the drama of disease and death. Even if I did not know them very well, they came to see me, at least when I fell ill, or when my disease worsened.

Many otherwise stalwart friends do not know how to handle

the situation when they first come to cheer you up. Leonard Probst advised them not to talk about his mental state because they felt they were expected to. This attitude he said, comes from embarrassment or possible guilt at avoiding cancer, and often deadens the conversation and led him to thinking about himself, which can be depressing.

Others disagree with him, and I am on their side. Writing to *The New York Times*, one woman said the very act of explaining her disease diminished it and reassured everyone; another that sharing what's on a patient's mind gave him a chance to unburden himself a bit and feel better for it. The list of hints for hospital visitors in chapter three sums it up. It's best to be caring, casual, straightforward, and to take your cues from the patient as to how much he wants to unburden himself. Don't shy away from him. Look him—or her—in the eye!

My favorite friends: the teenage boys who visited a patient pal at Sloan-Kettering. The youngster was blue; chemotherapy had caused his hair to fall out and left him feeling odd. But when he saw his friends he cheered up. They had shaved their heads completely and were as bald as he.

CHAPTER 7

ME AND JOHN CHANCELLOR

It was October, a lovely time of the year in Washington, D.C. I was resting in bed, getting over my mastectomy operation. I was feeling pretty good. My recovery had been speedy. The doctors had told me they felt optimistic about my future.

Then I turned on the Nightly News. John Chancellor was talking about Betty Ford's recent operation. "Breast cancer," he reported, "is a killer," and proceeded to prove it with statistics. There would be 89,000 new cases that year of 1974 and 32,500 women would die of the disease, the most common form of death for women between the ages of 31 and 55.

The newsman had turned cancer specialist minus white coat and stethescope. From him, and from his colleagues in all the media, I learned that nine out of ten biopsies turn out to be benign. For those of us who were not so lucky, for those with malignant biopsies, the chances for survival after five years were about 75 percent (65 percent after ten years) if there is no spread to the axillary (armpit) lymph nodes, but only 30 percent (25 percent after ten years) if there was such a spread.

Something about the blunt cool way this information was presented by someone I didn't even know started me thinking, for perhaps the first time, that one of the unlucky 25 percent could just happen to be me. It was a dark thought. As a J.D. Salinger hero once put it, "it didn't make me feel too gorgeous."

And I blamed John Chancellor and Co. for bringing it to me, without regard for my feelings or sensitivities. This was not quite fair, of course. Common sense and experience told me the messengers should not be blamed for the message. It also told me it could have been brought more tactfully.

I do not think anyone has given much thought to how cancer news affects us patients. There are numerous examples of this. On the one end of the scale, my son Jeremy sends me a clipping from *Newsweek* headlined: "ICY AID FOR CANCER VIC-TIMS." It reports a new promising technique to spare patients taking chemotherapy the indignity of hair loss. Nurses at the University of Arizona fashioned ice packs to cool the scalps of cancer "victims" while Adriamycin was being administered. This prevented their hair follicles from absorbing the drug, and 70 percent of the patients retained most of their hair.

I am on Adriamycin and losing my hair. I rush to my oncologist, asking for an ice pack. He nixes the idea. Breast cancer patients can suffer metastases to the scalp; he sees no reason for making the effort I'm making and then not having the drugs reach potentially malignant sites for the sake of cosmetics. I agree. I am disappointed, but nothing is lost.

At the other end of the scale, *The Washington Post* last fall front-pages a sensational headline, "Experimental Drugs: Death in the Search for Cures." Two young investigative reporters had begun a series in which they detailed the gruesome effects of so-called Phase I or experimental anticancer drugs. As the week wore on, I got more and more nervous about the articles because the reporters did not seem to distinguish sufficiently between experimental drugs, which are given only when standard therapies have failed, and routine chemotherapy, with its nuisance-like, but bearable (for most people) side effects.

I was right to be nervous. As Sister Rosemary told me, when she described the negative effect these articles had on New York area Sloan-Kettering patients, "Cancer patients find articles." Chemotherapy patients on the drug were furious, and they soon deluged *The Washington Post* with letters telling how chemo had helped them. According to my George Washington oncologist, Phil Cohen, those about to begin a chemo course felt fearful and dismayed. One of his patients refused treatment. The gung-ho articles, anxious to make points, right or wrong, about the administration of a small group of drugs to a small group of people desperate to save their lives had profoundly troubled a larger group of hanging-in cancer patients.

Dr. Cohen spoke of other dramatic examples of the power of news purveyors. After reading sensational reports of a new "discovery" in the newspapers, cancer patients have been known to arrive unannounced at treatment centers on stretchers and in wheelchairs. Even so, it seems to me that the main problem is that the vast majority of cancer "communicators" I meet or read about, usually public information people working for government or private medical groups, fail even to consider how to approach anxious patients tactfully and hopefully, or how to avoid misleading them. They tend to talk simply about how best to use the media to get their messages across.

A Ph.D. at one conference in the mid-1970s (on the Behavioral Dimensions of Cancer) detailed for his colleagues studies conducted on the results of a Public Broadcasting Children's Workshop called "Feeling Good"—a series, he explained, intended to motivate, not merely to inform. Whenever possible, he advised, use "multiple appeals," or "a cluster of program segments," to reinforce the message. Use attractive segments, or demonstrations of correct behavior, rather than fear appeals. Do not denigrate people by calling them names like "fatso." Be wary of easily interpreted songs and parody.

And so on. Health education in the mass media is a big business, with tens of millions of dollars spent on it each year. But even based on their own priorities, cancer communicators have not been notably successful. These priorities aim to reduce death and disease rates through prevention (the action one can take to minimize risks) and early detection and proper treatment (the action one can take once the disease rears its ugly head by responding promptly to the seven warning signs of cancer* and getting to the doctor).

We all know that millions of people, especially men, have been shocked into stopping smoking by the news that this habit can cause lung cancer. Similarly, many millions of women have been motivated to get PAP tests to detect early cervical cancer, for which treatment is almost 100 percent effective. Far fewer have been inspired by the media to practice breast self-examination to detect early breast cancer. An interesting study conducted for the National Cancer Institute's Office of Cancer Communications (through Porter, Novelli and Associates) found little information about cancer prevention and detection in stories mentioning cancer from top newspapers. Prevention was the major topic in only 3 percent of almost 1,500 news stories published during three months of 1980, reaching at least one-third of all Americans; detection and diagnosis were the major focus in another 3 percent.

Except for lung and breast cancer, the most common forms of the disease were not covered extensively in most of these stories. Although almost two out of three people could be saved if they used early detection measures like the "procto" examination for colo-rectal cancer, the most common form of cancer, it was mentioned in only 6 percent of the stories analyzed. Cancers associated with the female and male reproductive organs, which rank fourth and fifth, received minimal coverage (9 and 5 percent, respectively).

Most fascinating for me was the finding that communicators had not made much dent in public misconceptions about cancer. Information placing cancer in proper perspective was lacking.

* ● Change in bowel or bladder habits
 ● A sore that does not heal
 ● Unusual bleeding or discharge
 ● Thickening or lump in breast or elsewhere
 ● Indigestion or difficulty in swallowing
 ● Obvious change in wart or mole
 ● Nagging cough or hoarseness

The vast majority of the cancer news stories analyzed concerned "hard," breaking news. About 33 percent described carcinogens and other possible causes of the disease; almost 18 percent concerned treatment, notably Interferon; and 16 percent were about famous people suffering from cancer, like actor Steve McQueen or Connecticut Governor Ella Grasso. Six percent focused on quackery and Laetrile.

These results closely resembled those obtained from a similar study done by the same group in 1977, except that with the death of Hubert Humphrey there were less VIP stories. There had been little change in three years, though, of course, there has been long-run change since the time when obituaries never mentioned the word cancer (people used to die "after a long illness"). Most of the stories in the study still tended to reinforce negative public attitudes and misconceptions. Like the bumper sticker, they conveyed the impression that "Life Causes Cancer" or that cancer is invariably a fatal disease; you die with it, you do not live with it. Fewer than 5 percent of the stories analyzed described the coping resources or help available to the hanging-in patient; a few more gave the reader some insight into how to cope successfully, how to get information about a specific cancer, for instance, or the importance of maintaining a positive attitude.

Some additional analysis of headlines in the recent study added to the picture. Although the headline language was judged almost equally optimistic, pessimistic, and neutral, headlines about the causes of cancer (notably chemicals in cosmetics, household cleansers, or clothing) were especially likely to arouse fear.

Headlines for colo-rectal or stomach cancer stories were generally more fear-arousing and pessimistic than headlines for lung or breast cancer stories; maybe south-of-the-border stories about cancers attacking less spiritual parts of the body seem more shameful to people. Headlines for hormone treatment were generally most optimistic.

In a way, the fall of 1974 was a different time. It was the best of times and the worst of times to fall sick with breast cancer. Best, due to the guts of Betty Ford and, to a lesser extent a few months later, of Happy Rockefeller, who spoke out about their mastectomies and made the rest of us feel it was all right to do so; their approach also made us feel less freakish and in good company.

Worst, because these two ladies in public life opened the gates to an onerous, sometimes overwhelming, flood of information. Drive your car to the grocery store, radio on; sit down at the typewriter or beauty shop within earshot of a fellow member of the human race, and there it was. Try to live a normal life, advised the doctors. Forget it, work, play, practice coué, urged a friend over a bloody Mary.

Impossible. As the years have gone by and other public figures like Hubert Humphrey and Marvella Bayh have shared their troubles, it has continued to be so. Disease talk, especially cancer talk abounds, even if it is not the talk cancer communicators prefer. Some of the societal attitudes it highlights are difficult for patients, and possible future patients, to live with.

The first is inherent in the tone and architecture of the "cancer is a killer" stories. There is something in the blunt, tell-it-like-it-is way they are presented that reflects the common wisdom that *knowing all the news, whatever it may be, is "good" for you. Conversely, it is "weak" to try to avoid even a single cancer statistic inferring bad news, even if it helps deprive you of hope.*

I disagree. Hope, I repeat once again, is the essential ingredient. Without it, we patients can find no reason for struggling to survive; without it, we find it easy to give up and stay in bed. I have worked several times with the Hubert Humphreys. In the 1964 campaign, when the senator ran for the vice-presidency with Lyndon Johnson, I served on Muriel Humphrey's staff. Four or five of us were squeezed into the Humphrey den on Coquelin Terrace in nearby Maryland. When you got out your compact you were apt to powder someone else's nose. I had worked for the Humphreys before, traveling in Wisconsin with Muriel in 1960, but it was in 1964 that I got to know him.

Hubert Humphrey's reputation as a proponent of the politics

of joy was well deserved. He would come down in the morning, his hands raw from the previous day's campaign hand pumping. Just being around him made you feel exuberant. His optimism was contagious. When he went into the hospital at Memorial Sloan-Kettering Cancer Center some years later for a difficult operation, he strode around the corridors in his bathrobe, encouraging his fellow patients. The staff loved him.

If this man could be shaken by media cancer stories, anyone could. Yet this is exactly what happened. He had wanted to be open and truthful about his cancer in the modern, in *his*, fashion. He had been able to accept from his doctors information about the progress of his bladder disease beyond the perimeter of surgery, and his statistical chances of survival (a drop from 50 to 20 percent since there was lymph node involvement).

This same information anguished both patient and family when it appeared on television and in news stories, more pessimistic perhaps, since his was a bottom-of-the-body cancer. Bombarded by cold statistics, the patient, a man who had often engaged in sharp public debate with dignity and personal consideration, felt like a horse in the Belmont stakes. In the same way, Marvella Bayh cried, "I am *not* dying!" when she read and heard misinterpreted reports of the manner in which a doctor had told her she might have only a year to live, "I am living with the knowledge that I have cancer."

Of course most of us do not have to learn about our personal progress and statistical chances from the newspapers. But as far back as Camelot, they wondered what the king was doing that night. We tend to identify with the Betty Fords, Hubert Humphreys, and John Waynes, even the Shahs, when we learn they suffer our disease. We tend to get depressed, even to panic, when they get worse and to feel better when they improve. So there is a large unseen public out there, a public that reporters and editors seldom consider in telling VIP cancer stories.

Asked about their propensity for covering VIPs so extensively, editors and reporters will talk about their rights under the first [freedom of press and speech] amendment, and about their obligation to give the public information concerning presidents and world leaders. True of the Shah, and perhaps Senator Humphrey. But did a reporter really have the right to a courteous answer when he asked Betty Ford, as I heard him do at a Washington Press Club luncheon, how her cancer and alcoholism had affected her sex life?

The truth is that the ambience has changed. Time was when even a president's vital organs were entitled to some privacy. The press cooperated in minimizing Woodrow Wilson's semi-coma, and hiding the braces above Franklin D. Roosevelt's shoes. Now old standards have slipped, and new ones have not been devised. We seem to have lost our ability to strike a fair balance between the patient's right to privacy (whether to protect his future on the job, or in college, or his sensibilities) and society's legitimate need for health information.

In its zeal to satisfy our curiosity and increase the number of their readers and viewers, the media may be telling the public more than it needs to know. Certainly this public needs the latest information about the importance of avoiding carcinogens like smoke fumes or catching that breast lump or bone pain early, or getting the right treatment for it, or maintaining an optimistic outlook about it, and often the vehicle for this information is a story about a VIP. But it also needs to know that the truth about a person with cancer, even an important politician or movie star, is inevitably multidimensional and many faceted. Statistics are invariably arranged on a curve, some at one end, some at the other, most in the middle. Since every person responds differently to treatment, and medical knowledge remains imperfect, life-expectancy and other statistics may not fall into neat categories; you may turn out to be at either end of the curve.

As Sloan-Kettering's public affairs chief T. Gerald Delaney pointed out in the *Columbia Journalism Review* after the Humphrey hospitalization, doctors make flower arrangements with the facts, not only because it is easier to tell patients good news, but because there is a larger truth in the entirety of the arrangement, in the logic of the whole bouquet. News stories

108

seldom present patients with bouquets. It is the rare story that leads with good news, that the illness is well managed, the progress good, the outlook cheerful. It's the bad news, the stark, unmitigated facts, that command the headlines and make news. No wonder Ingrid Bergman chose to parry a reporter's question about her illness with, "One is not always well, but it is very personal and I don't want to talk about it."

Some reporters automatically invoke the first amendment when they are gently questioned about their right to probe in this way, whatever the situation. It's true that here in the United States the Constitution only protects patient-physician privacy through what the late Justice William Douglas called its "penumbras" (or shadows—the fourth, or search and seizure, and fifth, or self-incrimination, amendments). But medical ethics and federal and particularly state laws now protect some patient privacy to a limited extent.

What's more, legal scholars feel that though the first amendment gives reporters a helpful leg up in arguing for their privileges, the founding fathers intended it to protect the right to *publish* in the face of government autocracy. Not, in other words, to detail patients' bowel movements, or lack of them—information which might embarrass them and later endanger their prospects of getting insurance, or a job, or a college education, or even of recovering with zest and hope.

Susan Sontag, in *Illness as Metaphor*, has best publicized the second societal attitude that all of us hanging-in patients must live with. Despite the first attitude that it's good for you to know everything, there is a dark connotation attached to that about which you need to know. *Cancer, in fact, is a disreputable evil.*

Though cancer has been known to human beings for a long, long time (ancient Egyptian writings refer to tumors and primitive means of treatment—by knife), they have never come to regard it as ordinary. The passage of thousands of years has only mystified the disease process and those afflicted with it. Cancer, a word which comes from the Greek *karkinos* and the

109

Latin *cancer* (both meaning crab), has through the ages been associated with a sense of dread and evil. It is obscene in the original sense of the word: ill-omened, abominable, repugnant to the senses. A taboo surrounds people afflicted with cancer as it once surrounded people afflicted with tuberculosis. Nothing of that disgraceful taboo is attached to patients with cardiac disease, an illness implying merely weakness, trouble, mechanical failure.

What's more, cancer, the evil invincible predator, is not just a disease. In English, and other languages, the word has been applied figuratively to social, political, and other human enterprises. It was early regarded as a metaphor for sloth and idleness. "Sloth is a Cancer, eating up that Time, Princes should cultivate for Things sublime," wrote Edmund Ken in 1711. Susan Sontag cites many other examples of the use of the word cancer to describe corrosion of what was considered the social good: John Adams wrote in his diary in 1772 that "Venality, Servility and Prostitution spread like a cancer." Trotsky called Stalinism a cancer that must be burned out with a hot iron. Somewhat differently, D.H. Lawrence called masturbation "the deepest and most dangerous cancer of our civilization." And we all know how John Dean explained Watergate to Richard Nixon, "We have a cancer within—close to the Presidency—that's growing."

It used to be the more romantic passive disease tuberculosis, now it is cancer that secretly and ruthlessly invades and corrodes people and institutions. Every cancer patient carries around the baggage of cancer as a synonym, not only for death but for demoralization and devastation. To rectify the conception of the disease, argues Sontag, would make it less something to hide. It will remain so until, like tuberculosis, its etiology becomes clear and its treatment effective.

Implicit in these analogies, I heard Dr. Melvin J. Krant tell the 1981 American Cancer Society's National Conference on Human Values and Cancer, is that, "a good society as well as a good people must be on guard against this sneaky malevolent, infiltrative thing." A startling consequence is the question of contagion. Since mysterious forces can never really be understood, rational positions about communicatibility seldom relieve the deep doubt people harbor, which creates feelings about "being on guard" against cancer.

Oncologist Krant, a Professor of Medicine at the University of Massachusetts School of Medicine, feels that though open public quarantine of cancer patients no longer occurs, reported "clustering" of leukemias and other cancers, and news coverage of reports on virus particles relating to cancer, reinforce uncertainties about the communicable nature of the disease. He told the ACS meeting about a middle-aged couple in the hospital. The wife commented that she had stopped allowing sexual intercourse with her husband, who had advanced metastatic renal cancer. She knew, logically, she could not catch cancer "that way," but once in bed something else took over and she "couldn't do it." What's more she was furious when her married daughter (by a first marriage) questioned her "catching" cancer from her husband, but soon realized the daughter was only echoing her own sentiments.

No one knows the unhappy reputation of cancer and the rejecting behavior it evokes, even in settings of supposed acceptance and worth, better than the politicians. Golda Meir kept the knowledge of her disease secret for over a decade rather than risk sharing it with the public. In the dark of the night, she would go for her radiation treatments. She preferred this subterfuge to endangering her political fortunes and those of her government.

People sometimes do not take kindly to cancer patients as we saw in the last chapter, much less take the chance of electing them to high office. Though I have never experienced blatant shunning myself, I am a realist. I know that though the open use of the word cancer may be changing slowly, its implications for death and disaster may not be. I have heard about a prominent cancer center which advised its patients to hide their identification bracelets when they left the premises for a few hours, and about patients forced to eat off paper plates at home.

But I could hardly believe a news story a few years ago about a Maryland police captain who changed his officers' work schedule. The captain, who had been undergoing chemotherapy, came to his office to find a sign on the door saying "Danger, radioactivity," and to hear some of his men call him "Captain Chemo" and "glowhead."

Another pervasive attitude that haunts patients nowadays is *scapegoatism*. Very often, patients are made to feel they are at fault for falling and staying ill.

I was in George Washington University Medical Center, in the capital (put on the national map a few years later by its swift and successful treatment of President Ronald Reagan's gunshot wound). I was lying still, minding my own business, when a nurse came in to check on me. She was Indian, no credit to Mme. Ghandi.

"What's the matter with you?" she wanted to know.

I told her I had metastatic breast cancer, though she could have seen this on my chart.

"Why?" she wanted to know, and she persisted. She asked me if I had been to the doctor for checkups before I got cancer.

I told her I had been checked regularly every three months over a decade's time and had fallen sick with cancer anyway, but that did not stop her. When I had my mastectomy, why didn't I talk to the doctor about avoiding spread?

My patience was running out, but I replied weakly that I had talked to many specialists about avoiding spread. When she started muttering about "stage four," I told her that was enough; I would rather not discuss the matter with her any further.

Such crude tactlessness is grounded in absolute faith in the patient's ability to control her own medical destiny: if only you had obeyed the medical rules, you would be in the clear. Beyond this there are more subtle attitudes that inflict guilt on patients. There is the unafflicted man's perhaps unconscious feeling that we get what we deserve in this world, and there must be some justice in the patient's fate. Of course, if the patient brings the disease on herself, he protects himself from vulnerability to it. What's more, he can absolve himself from responsibility for helping. Unconsciously or not, we patients feel such attitudes particularly when they are reflected in media stories. If only we had lived *right!* If only we had jogged, or eaten in a nutrition-wise fashion, or enjoyed more emotional fulfillment. If only....

One friend of mine shrugged off my first metastasis. Like many people, he feels comfortable only if he can manipulate everything to fend off and control disease. He rides a bicycle to work. He eats a special bran cereal each morning. For me, he advised yoga. Yoga had helped him cure his lower-back pains, yoga was what I needed to cure my troubles. No matter that the doctor had told me to take it easy. Months later, when he heard Sloan-Kettering's judgment about my bone scans, he finally, reluctantly, accepted my illness.

People are always sending me clippings of stories stemming from a study done in Alameda County, California, by Dr. Lester Breslow and statistician Nedra Belloc. This study showed that if you followed seven old-fashioned simple rules, your chances of good health and longer life increase:

1. Don't smoke cigarettes;
2. If you drink alcohol, do so in moderation;
3. Eat breakfast;
4. Don't eat between meals;
5. Maintain weight;
6. Sleep seven or eight hours a day;
7. Exercise moderately.

There is little medical quarrel with rules one or two. But some doctors, including the distinguished Lewis Thomas, have pointed out that statistics demonstrating such rules don't tell us too much. It's the healthy people who are apt to be out there jogging. More important, admonitions about healthy living may not apply in individual cases, where a host of factors, including heredity and environment, play significant parts.

I know this is true. I followed the rules. I ate breakfast, gave up smoking, went to Weight Watchers, slept soundly, did moderate exercises for years at the Watergate Health Club, drank only "socially." Yet, as I have repeatedly pointed out, I developed cancer at about the same age as my grandmother and in the same pattern.

Stories about health-mongering rules tempt policy makers, of course, because advice is cheaper than modern treatment. It used to be that if your neighbor fell ill with cancer or heart disease (or anything else), he had to pay his own medical bills. Nowadays, we are increasingly responsible for each other's medical bills. And they are increasingly expensive. If enough insured Americans go into the hospital with lung cancer, your insurance premiums will rise. If they are covered by Medicaid, your taxes will rise.

The late Dr. Michael Halberstam, that ebullient and productive Washingtonian who lost his life when he courageously accosted a robber-murderer, spoke out repeatedly on this subject, believing it unfair to blame patients for their sickness and its cost. The health-oriented Robert Wood Johnson Foundation's president, Dr. David E. Rogers, has pointed out that when human beings are affected by something personally, they tend to seek out villains. If costs of health care rise too high, as indeed is the case, they now tend to blame the sick and unhealthy. They say we "overuse" medical care, or we do not use it appropriately. We either do not avail ourselves of regular preventive checkups, or conversely, we bring every ache and pain we suffer to the doctor.

We don't. Rogers argues that most people seem to use medical care quite sparingly. Few enjoy being poked and probed or enduring painful treatment and surgery. They go to the doctor when they are frightened, or in pain, or both. Whether their symptoms turn out to be signs of significant illness or not, they should not be considered trivial. Doctors should deliver reassurance as part of good medicine.

Amen. There *are* a few hypochondriacs. And as I have observed (chapter 3) lonely people especially find hospitalization an attention-grabbing, exciting event. They are far fewer, however, than the people who put off going for treatment and are anxious to be sprung from the hospital. Studies of prepaid medical programs bear this out.

Oncologist Melvin Krant observes that it is the tension between wanting things to look good on the one hand and being direct and realistic on the other that causes pain for hanging-in patients.

We may want to get on with the business of living and take a breather from being "sick." But some of us, and some even loving attentive family members, may feel confused, lonely, and angry when we read and hear news that makes us feel we are somehow to blame for our illness.

The "if you had only jogged" stories are not quite as invidious as the mismanaged emotions "if you had only been happy" ones discussed in chapter 5. But whatever the accusation, it does not help to react like the pitiful woman mentioned at the end of that chapter, weeping because she could not get her act together and get a leg up on her cancer, as the people in a magazine article she had picked up in the supermarket supposedly had done.

Better to insist that our disease is just that, a disease for which the cause or causes are still, unfortunately, murky. That is the healthiest way of hanging in.

CHAPTER 8

MONEY: THE NEVER-NEVER ITEM

Estelle Scott (not her real name) sits heavily on the couch she has turned into a bed in her small, dark southeast Washington living room. She turns off the afternoon television "story" when I come in and shushes three barking hound dogs. A portable commode sits awkwardly to the side of the couch. Two paintings of strong black faces decorate the drab wall behind it.

Mrs. Scott, a patient at D.C. General Hospital, the capital's public "hospital of last resort" on whose governing commission I serve, suffers the same disease as I, metastatic breast cancer. She is only a few years older, and, in major ways, her treatment has resembled mine: surgery, followed by radiation, chemotherapy, and hormone therapy.

But our hanging-in lives seem very different. Hers is narrower, more constricted. She cooks and cares for herself, yet rarely gets out, venturing regularly only up the block to the Safeway, and every other Saturday to the neighborhood beauty shop. A Literary Guild member, she says she loves to read and loves to get out and go places. She tells her friends, "I'll be ready to go when you get here." But she is dependent on them to "go," for her arthritic hips make it difficult to climb bus steps and her, or more precisely her late husband's, old car is up on blocks in the back yard waiting for money to fix it.

Though D.C. General offers care regardless of ability to pay, Mrs. Scott can not be considered poor. She no longer wants to work and does not need to. A retired file clerk and army widow, she draws two government pensions amounting to just over $1,000 a month. Her small house is almost paid for and cousins, a couple and three children, who moved in at her request after she fell ill, crowd the house but share some expenses. Most important, she is part of a small minority (3½–5 percent) of D.C. General patients who are covered, as I am, by commercial or Blue Cross/Blue Shield health insurance (she by Aetna, I by Blue Cross/Blue Shield). We are both part of the fortunate three-fourths of privately insured Americans who have major medical coverage.

On a routine visit to a D.C. General Hospital clinic for a blood pressure checkup in June of 1978, Mrs. Scott switched gears and headed for the Emergency Room. There she called the doctor's attention to a breast that had troubled her for over six months and that had now abcessed. Straightaway, he admitted her into the hospital for a mastectomy.

Since then, she has run up medical bills worthy of the term "catastrophic illness." She is not sure how much six weeks of radiotherapy and almost a year of chemotherapy and other subsequent outpatient care cost her out-of-pocket. She just pays each time she visits the clinic, then sends her receipts to Aetna for reimbursement, now $68 per visit every three months. She does know she got a $38,836 bill covering, as she understands it, her two hospital stays, for the mastectomy, and later, for a slow-healing, ulcerated radiation burn on her hip. She paid a small portion of this, less than $1,000, and her insurance company picked up all but about $8,000 of the remainder.

The hospital billing people started to put Mrs. Scott on a local medical assistance supplementary program for the medically needy and went so far as to get her an assistance card. With this, they planned to pick up half the $8,000 she owed, and have her pay the rest. It didn't work out that way. Though she turned her house inside out, Estelle Scott simply could not find papers to document her income during her two hospital stays (specifically, the Veterans' Administration forms documenting her husband's benefit check). She did find an additional commercial group veterans' policy her husband had carried, but by the time she wrote to that company in Pennsylvania, she was too late. The year-long filing date for supplementary payment had passed.

It does not occur to her to hound the Veterans' Administration for duplicate forms or to argue with the Pennsylvania insurance company, explaining that no one had told her she was going to need supplemental payments. So she is paying off the $8,000, at $50 a month, probably for the rest of her life.

This does not cause her any real hardship. But the debt bothers her. If someone left her a half a million dollars, she would not change her treatment site and go to Sloan-Kettering, like me; she is well satisfied with D.C. General, except for the fact that its computers continue routinely to bill her each month for over $32,000, all but $8,000 of which has long since been paid. Instead, she would pay off her hospital bill. Then she would pay the little she still owes on her house and take a long cruise, something she has always wanted to do. In other words, she'd buy herself some "quality" time.

Whether it's a matter of education, or cultural experience, or some mystery of sociologic stratification, Estelle Scott not only hangs in helped by fewer amenities than I, but she hangs in more passively. She still wears no prosthesis, more than three and a half years after her mastectomy. At the time of surgery she felt she could not afford one, and by the time she learned her insurance could cover the cost, she felt it was too late; she was used to going without one anyway.

She does not blame doctors, or other hospital staff, or even the larger society for anything substantial in her cancer experience: for public hospital clinic medicine that failed to provide her with a primary-care doctor of her own, who might have increased her chances by getting her into treatment faster; for

119

her radiation burn; for the lack of conveniences when she was in the hospital—no privacy (she had three roommates last time in, no private bathroom), no telephone, no television set (she had to bring her own; now the hospital has installed more semiprivate rooms, telephones, and TVs).

She blames herself for everything: delaying over six months before calling her disease to the doctor's attention; being too fat (she weighed as much as 260 pounds before she went on a diet recently) and not holding up her stomach as instructed when her hip was radiated so that she suffered a burn; losing the papers that would have helped her pay the hospital. A cheerful soul, she suspected her illness was somehow meant to be.

Since she feels that way, and in addition is not very agile at maneuvering the health care system, or nonsystem, she has not come upon anyone since she left the hospital to help her use what resources it and others in the city offer for the difficult hanging-in process. Once, on a clinic visit, she talked with a hospital social worker. But this lady, probably exhausted from the long day's battle helping patients solve fundamental problems, and pleased to find someone who was at least insured, housed, clothed, and functioning, only told Mrs. Scott her own problems!

Money is the paper anamoly of the hanging-in culture, king in an economic never-never land. It reigns all important, yet singularly unimportant; unreal, yet real enough to affect the subtlest parts of our lives.

The medical market place differs from any other. Buyers rarely reach into their wallets, count their bills, and pay for a service directly. Instead, most sign forms documenting their doctor or hospital use; medical offices feed items about their care into a computer. Eventually, we patients receive either a bill or reams of incomprehensible computer printouts. If we are lucky and have enough time, we might be able to figure out what we owe and to whom, and what part of our costs insurance will pay, be it public or private. Since buyer and seller seldom face each other at the cash register or even discuss cost, both tend to

120

be less sensitive to price than they are when buying anything else, from house to holiday to stereo set.

What's more, we consumer-patients usually have very little to say about our medical services. Whether we buy a car or rent one or take a bus, we may choose among various brands and styles. When we consult a physician, he or she normally prescribes the health services we get, be they a computerized axial tomography (CAT) scan, expensive medicines, or by-pass heart surgery. Mrs. Scott might run up a $38,836 bill. I might run up bills, as I did in just one year, for almost $11,000. But hardly ever do either of us talk with our doctors about the price of alternative treatments. Though the cost of my second mastectomy in 1981 ($3,000 to the hospital; $1,500 to the surgeon) was more than twice that of my first in 1974 (almost $1,600 to the hospital; $450 to the surgeon), our discussions never centered on cost, but on which treatment might best prolong my life and sustain its quality.

What I want, and what every patient wants, is to get well, and if that is not possible, to hang in well. If new esoteric cures take shape, we want them; we *will* have them. What the physicians can supply creates demand; price has little to do with it. Someone, we trust, will pick up most of the bill, be it insurance company or taxpayer.

All we can do is get down on our knees every night and thank the powers that be if we have insurance and it covers us adequately, like another hanging-in patient I know. Marcia Wilson suffered Hodgkin's disease at the age of twenty three. She has a mind for figures and has spent quite a bit of time going over her medical bills. She estimates that her treatment, including six hospital stays in 1976 and 1977, cost over $18,300; Blue Cross/Blue Shield picked up the tab. In addition, she had six weeks of radiation and six months of chemotherapy for which she does not have complete records.

Playing with her calculator, she once estimated the medical cost of her two-year illness at between $20,000 and $25,000, and the *total* cost, including items as diverse as chemotherapy, wigs, transportation to Sloan-Kettering for one hospitalization,

121

'and the amount she did not earn when she was out of her Justice Department job, at $75,000. A study of 364 terminal cancer patients done in 1981 for the Department of Health and Human Services showed that their last six months of care averaged $10,912. But Susan Walker, an American Cancer Society social worker in Washington, says that in 1982, $10,000 is a drop in the bucket for a long-term patient. You can hardly get a hospitalization for that; she's used to seeing $48,000 or $50,000 medical bills. What do people who are uninsured, either all or part of the time, some 34 million Americans, do?

Money influences our hanging-in lives first, in subtle ways. For money, or more broadly, what money buys in the way of habits and lifestyle, seems to affect both who gets cancer in the first place (incidence), and how we do after we get it (survival).

Studies of cancer incidence are maddeningly complex and difficult to sort out; you can only glean clues from them as to cause and effect. But researchers have been finding for some time that certain population groups suffer more cancer than others.Since such groups in our pluralistic society have different average income levels and different styles in which they use that income, the implication, at least, is that income or money is involved in disease incidence.

According to a recent five-year National Cancer Institute study covering more than 10 percent of the population, for instance, cancer rates among black men are alarmingly high, 22 percent higher than among white men, although black women have slightly fewer cancers than white—and blacks as a group have lower average incomes than whites. Inner-city black men (in Washington), who have generally low incomes, suffer twice the amount of cancer of the esophagus as white men nationwide (esophageal cancer commonly strikes heavy smokers and drinkers and may be associated with diet, too).

Hispanics, regardless of income level, develop at least one-third less cancers than do other Americans, a difference that points primarily to cultural rather than income differences—for

122

medical scientists speculate that the reasons include a diet high in proteins but low in meat. So Hispanics' cancer rates may increase, as have those of other immigrants like the Japanese, as they become more like other Americans in lifestyle habits. Or they may not increase, if the difference is rooted primarily in genetics.

Dr. Susan Devesa, an NCI epidemiologist, has pioneered in trying to find out how income and education specifically affect two kinds of cancer. She found a strong positive association between income and education and breast cancer among over 19,000 white women: The more income and education they had, the more breast cancer. On the other hand, among a much smaller sample of black women she found a positive association with education but not with income: Money made less difference in incidence than did education.

It was the other way round with cervical cancer. Both income and education affected who got cancer among white and black women: The less money and schooling you had, the higher the risk. When Dr. Devesa removed socioeconomic factors from her computations, she cut black-white differences in breast cancer rates in half, and the excess risk of cervical cancer rates among black women was reduced by two-thirds.

Dr. Devesa speculates that it is not income or education in themselves that cause such differences, it is the way income and education affect a woman's life, which is really what most of the other incidence researchers tell us when they finger money only by implication as a cancer cause. A breast cancer patient's diet (which influences the hormone environment within her body) influences risk, and people with higher incomes and more education often eat richer foods than those with less, and so have higher risks. The finding that a black woman with more education had more chance of getting breast cancer than the black woman with less, may reflect the postponement of the birth of her first child to pursue her schooling; she is older, and at more risk, when she has her first child. Differences in sexual practices often associated with socioeconomic level—the number of sexual partners a woman has, for instance, and so the number of

123

viral infections she is exposed to—may affect her risk of contracting cervical cancer.

So we see that the role of money in who gets cancer is fuzzy. It becomes clearer when it comes to what happens to you *after* you fall ill.

Poor patients plainly fare worse than those with more money, often much worse. There are many reasons. Poor people usually have less access to medical care than their nonpoor counterparts. They perceive themselves to be in poorer health when they get into treatment and usually are. They go to the doctor's office less, are more likely to patronize emergency rooms and outpatient clinics than people who have more income, and have to travel longer to get there. When you don't feel well you are less likely to want to wait for the bus and travel bumpily to the clinic. So you delay going to the doctor or don't go at all.

We're beginning to get better statistics than we have had in the past about how Americans use health care. In a paper prepared for the President's Commission for the Study of Ethical Problems in Medicine and Biomedical and Behavioral Research, Johns Hopkins health economist Karen Davis reports that, in 1978, poor whites and blacks with no insurance, wherever they lived, were about twice as likely *not* to have seen a doctor over a two-year period as nonpoor white people with private insurance living in metropolitan areas. Only 3 percent of these nonpoor whites used hospital emergency rooms or outpatient departments as their usual source of care, as opposed to 36 percent of the poor blacks with no insurance in the same area. Thirteen percent of the same nonpoor whites traveled half an hour or more to get care, in contrast to 27 percent of the poor blacks. They generally perceived that they were almost twice as healthy, only 9 percent thought they suffered fair or poor health, in contrast to 17 percent of the poor blacks.

For us cancer patients, the stage (how far and how much the disease has spread from its original site) is very important. Medical scientists have known for some time that the stage of most cancers at initial treatment influences the time we survive. A 1976 National Cancer Institute report tells us that white patients had a 73 percent chance of surviving five years if they were diagnosed early, with localized (Stage I) disease, while they only had a 47 percent chance if their cancer had spread (to "regional," Stage II). In the same way, black patients with breast cancer had an 80 percent chance of surviving five years if their disease was diagnosed early (Stage I) in contrast to a 46 percent chance if it had spread to Stage II (regional, and it could spread to distant parts of the body—Stage III, lowering survival chances even further). Survival chances for many cancers have improved since the mid-seventies. But it's still better to be seen earlier, and indigent people are often first seen by the doctors at later stages.

Still, the University of Colorado Medical Center's Dr. John Berg, one of the few researchers to focus his attention on how socioeconomic status affects cancer patients, tells us that indigent patients with every type of cancer have poorer chances for survival than nonindigent, *regardless* of the stage of the cancer at initial treatment. Comparing patients treated in the same University of Iowa hospital by the same housestaff, Berg found that the indigent had higher death rates after diagnosis from causes other than cancer, as well as excess mortality not accounted for by stage difference. This was particularly true among patients with less lethal cancers who should have survived longer; instead their cancers occurred more often and earlier than those of patients with enough money.

The important thing here is that Dr. Berg's Iowa patients all received the same quality of care. So there have to be other reasons for such striking differences in their survival times he found as these: Indigent patients with cancer of the rectum survived a median time of 22 months, while private patients survived 48; indigent patients suffering nasopharynx cancers survived 12 months, private patients 31.

Continuing his study of cancer risks in Colorado, Berg compared the survival time of patients living in different census tracts and found again that people from high-income tracts did

125

better than those from low-income tracts. All in all, the results were similar to those of his previous study and to those of the small number of other such socioeconomic studies. Almost half of the "anglo" patients (45 percent) from high-income census tracts were alive after 5 years, but only a third (34 percent) of the poor patients survived that long. The poor had more cancers of poorer prognosis and less of good prognosis.

Dr. Berg postulates that "host differences" associated with poverty may account for such differences in our chances of survival. This means that there is a tendency for cancer cells to implant themselves in abnormal body tissue, in the connective tissue of malnourished people, for example, or in body tissues which have been weakened by alcohol, or heavy smoking, or generally poor health. If your body acts as a welcoming host to cancer cells because it has been damaged by something money might have helped you avoid, then lack of money lessens your chances for survival.

At the George Washington University Medical Center desk where I must present myself (sometimes without breakfast) whenever I am scheduled for a scan, or another test, or an outpatient biopsy, the admitting clerks do not even say "good morning." They don't ask for money—directly. Instead, they ask, "May I see your insurance card?"

If we hanging-in patients can be baffled by the subtle ways money affects our hanging-in lives, we are often even more confused by its everyday impact. So, indeed, is the larger society. Not that American health care managers are unconcerned about money; they are deeply concerned, as they should be. In 1980, we spent $247.2 billion on health care. (That's over 9 percent of our gross national product.)

If you look at cancer costs alone, the government's National Center for Health Statistics tells us that the national bill for neoplasms (malignant and nonmalignant tumors) was $7.2 billion as of last count in 1978, for the calendar year 1977, $5.7 billion for hospitals and $1.5 billion for physician's services. These are direct costs, dealing with prevention, diagnosis, and treatment, the kind of hospital and medical bills I ran up last year. If you include indirect costs, or the current value of the amount patients would have earned had their illness, disability, or death not caused them to miss work, the cost rose in 1977 to between $29 billion and $35 billion, depending on the rate by which economists computed it. Don't forget such costs continue to rise: The amount the American people had to spend on their total personal health care rose between 1977 and 1981 from $218 billion to $250 billion.

People in other industrialized countries seldom understand the way we try to meet these costs and assure health care. Once when I was abroad interviewing a Spanish health official, I mentioned that we had no one comprehensive national health insurance plan covering everyone in the United States, similar to those in European countries. I explained that we had such plans only for elderly people and for the very poor. He did not believe me. Surely such a situation could not prevail in the land of milk, honey, and computer chips! "What?" he asked, appalled, "Not even in the District of California? Not even in the District of Illinois?"

Not even in the District of California. Not even in the District of Illinois. What we do have, as you have probably learned as a hanging-in patient, is a patchwork of public and private programs that creak along haphazardly and somewhat expensively. If you happen not to fit into the category they were set up to cover, or if you do not know about them and are not sophisticated in using them, you can slip between the cracks.

Gail Wilensky, a senior economist at the National Center for Health Services Research, is uncovering some interesting facts about this patchwork, and your relation to it. Her agency has begun to analyze a survey of a sample of 40,000 people living in all parts of the country in 1977, probably one of the most comprehensive health insurance surveys ever done. This National Health Care Expenditures Study tells us that some 177.8 million people (or 83.9 percent) of the civilian noninstitutional population has full-time, year-round coverage. Some 34.2 million lacked such coverage, but only 18.2 million were completely uncovered all year; the other 16 percent had coverage part of the year. At any given time about 25 million were not covered.

Looking specifically at one of the biggest hanging-in groups, us several million cancer patients, Gail found that 8 percent are uninsured part of the year. Of this number, 4.5 percent are always uninsured (more about this later). The rest of us are covered by the following:

Medicare (38 percent), the federal program that provides hospital and medical insurance for people 65 years of age and over; as well as for some disabled and some kidney disease patients under 65;

Medicaid (7 percent) the federal-state program for Americans on welfare and for certain other categories or people— the poor aged (65 or older), the blind, the disabled, members of families with dependent children, and some other children.

Private insurance (49 percent) either Blue Cross/Blue Shield or commercial companies, whose policies range from those that cover bare hospital room and board charges to "major medical" plans, like mine, covering inpatient costs completely and all but 20 percent of most of my outpatient costs.

On paper this looks good, for everyone except the 8 percent of the hanging-in cancer patients who are uninsured, either all, or part of the time. But difficult problems can arise, though you enjoy, or think you enjoy, insurance protection.

In the first place, even if you are over 65 years of age* and, like almost all other elderly people throughout the United States, are covered year round by Medicare, this federal health insurance program pays only part, not all, of your health care expenses. Hospital insurance, or Part A, financed by social

*According to the National Health Care Expenditures Study, almost half of the cancer patients (48 percent) are 65 or older, 3 percent are under 18, and another 48 percent between 19 and 64 years of age; 71 percent are white and 29 percent other than white; 45 percent male and 55 percent female; 34 percent poor and low-income, 33 percent middle-income, and 30 percent high-income.

security payroll deductions, covers your inpatient hospital costs except for the first $260 in each benefit period (there are ninety days in a benefit period and patients have an additional life time reserve of sixty more days) as well as a small coinsurance fee, beginning on the sixty-first day you pay $65 per day ($130 a day if you are using your reserve). It also covers some of your posthospital care in a skilled nursing home up to 100 days (you pay $32.50 beginning on the twenty-first day) and an unlimited number of health visits (provided you are home bound and require skilled nursing care).

You can buy, if you wish, Medicare's Part B, a medical insurance program, financed now largely through general revenues. It is voluntary and requires low supplemental monthly payments of about $12. In return, it offers you some protection against doctor's costs, medical services like laboratory and x-ray tests, home health care services, ambulance and other outpatient services, and supplies, like hospital equipment for use at home. As in Part A, there is a deductible, which you must pay each year, and coinsurance: Medicare medical insurance now usually pays $4 out of each $5 of reasonable medical charges except for the first $75 in each calendar year. It does not cover costs for items you often need when you are older, such as outpatient drugs or custodial care, dentures, eyeglasses, or hearing aids.

Local Social Security offices can give you the latest details about Medicare. If you are 65 or older, you should check there, because the law and regulations change from time to time. As I write in early 1982, the administration has proposed cuts in Medicare along with other domestic programs, which may cause still higher deductibles and more coinsurance.

If you are under 65, you still might want to check to see if you are eligible for other Medicare benefits. If you are totally disabled and cannot do any kind of work, you may be eligible for monthly cash Social Security disability benefits (your disability must be expected to last a year or more). These cash benefits can begin no earlier than the sixth month of your total disability. After you have been collecting cash benefits for twenty four months, you will be eligible for Medicare. And if you are suffering from kidney disease, you may be entitled to extensive benefits.

Medicaid, the federal-state assistance plan, offers many more benefits than Medicare to hanging-in patients. But it is available to you only if you are a member of certain groups of needy and low-income people. Every state offers some Medicaid services* (and some have supplementary insurance programs of their own for those who don't fit into Medicaid slots, like the one that Mrs. Scott hoped to use in Washington, D.C.). The various states design their own programs within federal guidelines.

Consequently, these programs vary from state to state. You can check on the details in your state at your local welfare or public assistance office. Generally, Medicaid pays at least basics, like inpatient hospital care, outpatient hospital services, other laboratory and x-ray services, skilled nursing and doctor services. In many states it pays for more: prescribed drugs, dental care, eyeglasses, or nursing homes. What's more, Medicaid can pay what Medicare does not pay for people eligible for both programs and can pick up their Medicare deductibles and coinsurances.

One important thing to check on is Medicaid's "spend down" provision. Many hanging-in patients don't know about this, but if your income and your resources become so depleted that you can be considered medically indigent, you can *become* eligible for Medicaid (that is probably why a mere 4.5 percent of us cancer patients are totally uninsured all the time). The rules vary from state to state, but generally you must have depleted almost all your liquid assets to be considered medically indigent.

Using a special fund to help patients with their medical expenses, the local American Cancer Society division has helped a man here in Washington, let's call him Mr. Kemper, who is hanging in with a nasty neck cancer. He must change

*Except Arizona, which plans to begin an experimental program in the fall of 1982.

130

dressings on his neck three times a day. These are expensive, and he is too sick to work, his savings have sunk lower than $2,500 and his income lower than $285 a month. He's about to go on Medicaid. Mr. Kemper, a proud man, who has held important jobs, does not want to accept public assistance, but he must because the insurance his employer helped pay for when he was working stopped when he was forced to retire, and he could no longer afford it.

Mr. Kemper's is not a rare case. You can loose, or leave your job; you can divorce or separate; you can travel away from home—and you can find yourselves ill and without insurance. A Virginia oncologist told me about a patient of hers who had lost her insurance when she accompanied her husband to Venezuela for a period. The doctor told me she found herself treating this patient differently from others who were insured, omitting, for example, expensive scans she thought should really be done. When I asked her about her attitude in such a case, she answered, "I skimp, and pray that she finds her way back into the system."

How can you find your way "back into the system"? What do you do if you are too young for Medicare, not needy enough for Medicaid (and unwilling to "spend down" your resources to qualify for it), or for some other reason, find yourself uninsured?

One thing you can do, as a health insurance expert put it, is "run for cover." This means that you try as hard as you possibly can to get a job, any job, where you would be eligible for group insurance coverage. It's not likely that you would be able to afford or get individual insurance at this point, particularly when you are already sick (and it's not nearly as good a buy anyway, that's why fewer people buy it). Put your pride on the shelf; the job itself is not your goal, it's the health insurance coverage the job brings with it. You need this until you can get on your feet again, and you might find it where you least expected, for example in an agency employing temporary office workers sent out by the day.

If you are too ill for work, even part time, you should check to

131

see whether any of the organizations or associations you belong to have group health insurance plans. Some of the professional and fraternal organizations, farm groups, veterans groups, groups like Hadassah, offer excellent plans, others are more limited. If I were not covered by my husband's Blue Cross/Blue Shield insurance I'd buy into the Washington Independent Writers group policy, but I'd have to wait for an open enrollment period, which occurs only at a certain time of year.

If you do not belong to such an organization, try to find one to join. Go to your public library and ask for a book listing trade, professional, and other associations. In those long lists, you may find a suitable organization. Remember, when you get in touch with its staff, to ask for its health insurance plan details. Compare plans. Shop for the best possible deal. Watch for clauses that exclude coverage of "pre-existing conditions," or that have long waiting periods before coverage can begin, or that ask for a "health statement" or physical examinations that can exclude you from important coverage.

Sometimes insurance agents can be helpful in putting together groups of small business people, for instance. Independent agents who did not sell you your policy can be helpful too, if you question them thoroughly and go over plans with them. Acquainting you with the fine print in your policy will prevent the unpleasant surprise you could be in for if you think you are fully insured and fall ill, only to find you are not fully protected because you do not have "major medical" or catastrophic coverage. More than three-fourths of privately insured people, the National Health Expenditures Study tells us, do have major medical coverage.

A fourth do not. This means their policies may not cover "ancillary charges" like radiology and lab fees. Or they do not pick up doctor fees or the cost of medicines, or they place an unrealistic dollar "cap" on coverage. As the old joke goes, a man fell out of a skyscraper window, but his health insurance only covered him to the twentieth floor; for the rest of the way down, he was on his own.

By contrast, major medical policies like my own High Option

Blue Cross/Blue Shield plan, cover us all the way down or up as the case may be: ancillary charges, in fact everything in the hospital, a major part of out-of-the-hospital doctor and drug costs, and virtually no dollar limit. Like Marcia Wilson, I am thankful for it, even when its premiums rise. With it, my costs are manageable. Without it, they would not be.

As we will see further in the next chapter, it would be difficult for us hanging-in patients to buy more insurance once we actually are ill. Years ago when I was first sick, I innocently thought of getting additional health insurance and chatted with an aggressive young salesman.

"By the way," he asked me, "have you had any major operations?"

"Are you kidding?" I said, "that's why I'm talking with you."

"A hysterectomy?"

"No, a mastectomy."

"I'll call you back."

He never did.

This is true even of so-called "cancer" or "dread disease" policies offered the public, of which the experts have been highly critical. A House of Representatives Select Committee on Aging, chaired by Congressman Claude Pepper, recently observed that these "dread disease" policies are "very limited in value" and there are significant abuses in their marketing. Some only cover "definitive cancer treatment," leaving the patient alone to deal with ailments or complications of this treatment, diagnosis, pathology reports, or rehabilitation.

Many communities have resources you might not know are available to you. For example, the doors of public general hospitals like D.C. General or Grady Hospital in Atlanta are open whether or not you are uninsured and can be considered "medically indigent." Using local tax dollars, these hospitals can provide care that is often as good as that in some community hospitals.

The catch here is that though many institutions may call themselves "public" or "county" hospitals, they are not truly for the whole public. Some do not accept you if you are on Medicaid, much less if you have no insurance at all. Figures are hard to come by, but out of some 1900 nonfederal short-stay hospitals, it's safe to say only that roughly 90 public general hospitals serving 63 of the country's 100 largest cities accept all comers. And public hospitals are closing as tax dollars are squeezed and costs skyrocket. Between 1950 and 1980 the total number of local public hospital beds (city, county, and special authority) fell from just under 41,000 to just over 25,000.

But check out your local public hospital. The social workers there, as well as in private community hospitals, are good sources of information. So are the workers staffing local social services offices. Other programs you should ask about:

- Hospitals that received construction funding under the Hill-Burton Act have to give a certain amount of free care each year for a limited number of years. If you have slipped between all the cracks, your hospital might be able to cover your care under its "Hill-Burton obligation."
- Major medical centers around the country carry out research programs that involve patient treatment, often federally funded clinical trials. If your disease is one of those under study, you may be eligible for such trials, and the free treatment they involve. My friend, the Judge who has twice had open heart surgery, was referred by his doctor to such a program at the National Institute of Health's Clinical Center. So he has gotten both his new heart valves free of charge!

Finally, many voluntary organizations can help hanging-in patients with costs their insurance does not cover. In Washington, the American Cancer Society helps people pay for a variety of costs—transportation to hospitals and clinics (which can run high over the long run), or liquid food supplements, or sickroom equipment, or homemaker service. One ill, resentful mother had a great deal of trouble with her son. He moved around, living now with a grandmother, now with an aunt. When these people died, and he had to return to his ill mother, the ACS picked up the cost of his short-term counseling.

George Washington University Medical Center social workers have put out 26 pages describing who offers what to cancer patients in Washington, D.C., whether it's insurance, Meals on Wheels, Home or Hospice care, wheelchairs, or transportation. One frustrated man wrote in *The Wall Street Journal* in the summer of 1981 about his experiences trying to get such services for his mother, who had arrived fatally sick with bone cancer to live with him. As his family became more centered on his mother, its life together deteriorated; a son could not study with all the arguing, his wife had to keep rushing home from work to care for her and take her this place or that.

Though he tried valiantly to get help in the shape of home-care workers, health aides, meals, cabs, day-care centers, and others, he reported he was always put off with the question, "Is she on Medicaid?" The family managed to patch together services that cost "a fortune" and obtained less than what others, who "had the foresight to be paupers" were getting for free. Don't expect to hear his voice raised to save Medicaid, he wrote, a program whose "lavish benefits" he helps pay, but from which he is excluded.

That point of view reflects the fact that an increasing number of hanging-in patients and their families now have to pay a surprisingly large part of their incomes out-of-pocket to cover medical expenditures. The new National Health Care Expenditures Study shows that 7 percent of cancer patients and their families are paying between 10 and 20 percent of their income out-of-pocket and another 7 percent *over* 20 percent. That's a lot of income.

But Laverne Madancy, the Washington, D.C. American Cancer Society services chief, has a different view. She reports that with Medicaid on the scene, and D.C. General Hospital as a back up, her group has not had to help poor patients cover their medical expenses. Instead, it has been able to use its special medical services fund for near-poor patients who do not qualify for Medicaid. Very seldom does it have to step in to help anyone with unaffordable surgery; most of its funds go for medically related expenses, like Mr. Kemper's dressings or liquid food sup-

135

plements or transportation to care. Laverne's voice is raised against proposed Medicaid cuts. She wonders what will happen to hanging-in patients when and if they are made.

What it seems to boil down to is this: When it comes to high medical technology, money is scarcely visible; the health care system, or nonsystem, operates in a fairly egalitarian fashion, rarely denying you a delicate operation or intricate scan, though as we saw in the case of the Virginia oncologist, it can ration these things when insurances are lacking.

When it comes to health care before or after the high technology—to preventive care, or rehabilitation, or to medically connected amenities like your own private doctors or less waiting to see them, or even a few necessities like medical dressings—then it's a different story, and some hanging-in patients without adequate insurance, for whatever reason, begin to pay large parts of their income out-of-pocket. Money becomes highly visible. It begins to buy privilege, and its offshoot, a more accomplished lifestyle with the ability to thread your way through the system, insures it.

CHAPTER 9

WORK

When "Captain Chemo" found a dead rat in his car, and later, a pile of garbage in his parking space, he did not tell his superiors. He thought his men at the Wheaton-Glenmont district police station in southern Maryland were protesting his switching them from a four- to a five-day work schedule.

But when he began to receive threatening phone calls at home, and when his wife got a midnight call in which a man, taunting her about her husband's cancer and chemotherapy, shouted obscenities at her, he did report the harassment.

Another Maryland story: Greg Walters tried to enlist in the Marines. Despite help from his parents, his senator, and his doctors who had treated him for a rare form of lymphoma, he did not make it.

The Marine Corps turned him down because he had not been "symptom free" for five years. Tears came to his eyes when the Marines landed in Cuba, at Guantanamo Bay. He felt fit; he wanted to be there.

Ours is a work-oriented culture; our adult lives center about our jobs. Work roots deeply in our society. It establishes our sense of worth, our identity.

Work, as Studs Terkel puts it in his important book *Working*, is about a search "for daily meaning as well as daily bread, for recognition as well as cash, for astonishment rather than torpor; in short, for a sort of life rather than a Monday through Friday sort of dying." In the United States especially, we feel we should earn by our labor for ourselves and our dependents. Our ethic suspects idleness: We say people are "poor but honest"; we suspect "welfare fraud." We tend to measure personal adequacy by the economic independence gained from work. Like Freud, we consider *lieben und arbeiten* (love and work) the two great moving impulses.

In this setting the hanging-in patient can be severely handicapped. As Jon, a forty-two-year-old bookkeeper with a colostomy told Frances Lomas Feldman and her researchers: "I received a death sentence twice, once when my doctor told me I have cancer, then when my boss asked me to quit because the cancer would upset my fellow workers. Except for my wife, that job was my whole world." Dr. Feldman, a professor of social work at the University of Southern California, is the author of a remarkable three-volume study of work and cancer health histories, done under the auspices of her state's American Cancer Society Division.

I have not, to my knowledge, experienced work discrimination due to my illness. In fact I have had a few positive experiences. For several years, while I was executive director of a small national organization, the National Commission on Confidentiality of Health Records, my largely doctor board of directors extended themselves to accommodate my hospitalizations and my half-time schedule (true, they got a good bargain: They paid me half time, and I usually worked three-quarters time, at least).

Later, I lucked in with my colleagues at the Department of Education. When Liz Carpenter, whom I had known as a Washington journalist and White House Press Secretary, called to ask me to take a speech writing job, I hesitated, knowing she is the kind of person who goes at 75,000 miles an hour and has little sympathy for those who drop by the wayside.

"But Liz," I said, "I've been sick."

"That's all right," she answered, "you're better now."

The Secretary of Education, Shirley Hufstedler, was a model employer too, solicitous, but not overly so. I shall always remember her telling me on a trip to Barnard College, that she wanted me to do just what I felt like doing, and no more. I appreciated that.

There were little things, too. The way my staff treated me at the Commission, matter-of-factly, but kindly enough to make sure I was comfortable. The way my office mate at the crowded Ed Department, long-time reporter and friend Isabelle Shelton, responded when my back hurt from typing: She offered to type my manuscripts, even when she was swamped herself.

But I had read about Captain Chemo and Greg Walters, and I knew that job discrimination against hanging-in patients existed. So I was pleased to hear the scholarly Dr. Feldman at a conference, and to know about her thorough study of the experiences and perceptions of some 277 work-able cancer patients, white collar workers, blue collar workers, and young people. Not only did the Feldman researchers interview these patients in depth, but their families, employers, doctors, and school personnel, along with additional groups of similar patients. There's a lot of experience reflected in the Feldman volumes, and a lot of points of view.

What's more, Dr. Feldman's governing factor in choosing her samples of clinically cured cancer patients was "the likelihood of prime employability" because of age, education, and ability. She reasoned that if these highly employable workers met with discrimination, those with lower qualifications would encounter even more difficulty in finding and holding work. Moreover, the studies were done in California, which stands out among the states for having a law which specifically forbids employment discrimination against people with "any health impairment related to or associated with cancer, for which a person has been rehabilitated or cured, based on competent medical evidence" (The Siegler Bill, an amendment to the state's Fair Employment Practices Code, which went into effect on January 1,

139

1976, shortly before the first Feldman study was published). I reasoned that if employment discrimination takes place in California, with its heightened sensitivity to the issue, the likelihood is that it takes place to an even greater degree in other states.

The Feldman studies tell us that the hanging-in patient's experience in the work place is not entirely gloomy. Far from it. Patients in all three of the studies had positive experiences, which at times outweighed the negative—white collar workers with head/neck, colo-rectal and breast cancer; blue collar workers with the same diseases; and young workers thirteen- to twenty-three-years-old at the time of their diagnosis (sixteen to twenty-nine at the time of the interviews), with cancers more common to their age group, such as Hodgkin's disease and other lymphomas, leukemias, bones/soft tissue, and thyroid.

This was true when the hanging-in patients looked for jobs, and, later, when they went back to work, or school. Some slipped easily back into full or part-time jobs. Some talked about coworkers who were "marvelous," about helpful supervisors and friends who, like my friend Isabelle, pitched in to help them with strenuous tasks. For this reason, as a breast cancer patient put it, "as time went on, I didn't feel that I was so different from other women." Added an ironworker, "I'm feeling desperate when I'm not working. I can't lean over and die at my age (44). So I've *had* two bouts! I'll be back at my job soon; they're holding it for me."

Feeling desperate when I'm not working. An overriding theme of the interviews was that work is held in high esteem; the drive is to get and hold a job. Over and over, hanging-in patients of all races and ethnic groups try to demonstrate to themselves and others that they are still useful, able to take care of themselves and to retain mastery over their lives in spite of disease. Appreciating, but sometimes resenting solicitous offers of help, the workers seek to carry their own weight, to gain and hold respect, to prove their stamina, and to show that

140

cancer had not impaired their function. A high proportion of the head and neck white collar workers with "obvious" results of cancer got jobs that put them in the public eye, as well as supervisory positions. "Lost chord" patients took jobs where they had to project their voices, which must have caused them pain.

That this is not bravado is shown in what kind of workers these hanging-in patients were. They worked harder, faster, better than other people. They performed stressful tasks, and were not poor risks. They were rarely absent. Most were away from work only eight or nine weeks at the time of the diagnosis and initial treatment. Subsequently, less than a fifth of the white collar workers and more than half the blue collar workers were not absent at all; nearly half of the young people were absent from work or school fewer than seven days.

Obviously, the hanging-in patients not only needed to work but liked to and were good at it, "My boss took one look at me and said, 'Well, you don't look quite the same. Get busy; I've been waiting for you.' He needn't have kept me. I'd been with him for six months, and seeing my changed appearance must have been a shock. But I've had advances in salary and responsibility."

That reminds me of Linda Eckley, the feisty secretary I've mentioned before. After her mastectomy, her doctor told her she would not last more than two or three months, and she responded, "You must be talking to someone else." She showed the same stamina on the job, where she says, "I work for wonderful people." Her boss sent her to his own doctor for a second opinion, and after later treatment for a brain tumor, asked his wife to take her shopping for a couch so she could nap after lunch. They got the couch, but Linda has been too busy working to nap.

But the news from the work place is not rosy, on the whole. There are some significant minuses emerging from the Feldman study statistics. Most of the men and women interviewed were working full time, or part time, or in school. But a good portion of them were unable to find the work they wanted or had had a job application turned down because of their history of cancer.

"I lost my job right after the leukemia was found," one of the young respondents explained. "You name it; I applied for it." He added that whereas it used to take him less than a day or so to find jobs, it took him "four months of lying" to get his present one. Generally, much greater job-hunting effort had to be made than before the diagnosis; the young workers' anxiety mounted as they looked, and it's no wonder. Forty-five percent of them were convinced that cancer was the reason for their failure to obtain jobs. Nearly three-fourths of these claimed they were told this was the reason.

The older people had trouble, too. They easily spotted clues as to why this was so. One person was asked to use a pencil instead of a pen in a public employment office; pencils are easier to discard! Thirteen percent of the white collar workers were unemployed or working less than full time; 22 percent had had at least one job application turned down because of cancer history. Twenty-three percent of the blue collar men and women had either left their precancer employer or been rejected for at least one other job because of their cancer histories.

Of course the former patients worried as to whether to tell prospective employers about their illness. ("Sometimes I wake up at night and worry if they should find out!") Of course, too, some may inadvertently have sent out signals during interviews that they were unsure they could keep to a job schedule or do a certain job. One woman with a mastectomy kept telling her employer her troubles only to be upset when she was dismissed. Similarly, a man with a colostomy brought up his toileting needs several times during an interview and did not get the job.

Still, the general "can-do" theme threaded throughout their troubles. Said a lithographic stripper, "I went back to work a month earlier than the doctor advised me, but I did it gradually ... I wanted to get back on the job. I take a lot of pride in my work, and I'm one of the most experienced men in the company."

Despite such insistence that they could carry their own

weight, the unemployed and less-than-full-time blue collar workers showed a slightly different pattern than the teachers, nurses, and other white collar people who were unable to find work. For one thing, most of them were physically unable to pursue their customary strenuous occupations, while the white collar men and women could have done the jobs they applied for.

For another, they were, by and large, more philosophic, more accepting of what they found in the work place. They were less vocal and reacted less strongly to discrimination. A young policeman who had lost a testicle to cancer, for instance, interpreted the ribbing he got from his fellow officers as "normal," friendly, and affectionate interest in him; he developed a roster of replies to draw on when he heard their ribald comments.

When they returned to work, 54 percent of the white collar workers and 84 percent of the blue collar workers had one or more problems related to the cancer experience. Thirty-five percent of the latter viewed the problems as discriminatory. There were a tremendous variety of these problems; the blue collar workers alone had 37 different kinds.

Many had to do with the job itself. Some were natural problems, like the special effort that had to be made to find time to go for treatment (several changed to the night shift or otherwise arranged their hours so they would not have to be absent).

Some workers reported they received no salary advances when colleagues did, their health benefits were reduced, they were excluded from group health plans, or declared ineligible for group life insurance, or ineligible for a period of five to eight years for income-replacement disability. One man said that his insurance was cancelled on the automobile he needed to get himself and his tools to work.

A woman grew depressed because she could not project her voice on the job, "They took advantage of me and demoted me." Several foremen were demoted because their impaired speech made it difficult for them to convey orders and led subordinates and colleagues to ridicule them. Blue collar workers had an additional problem. They often were employed on an hourly wage basis, and even if they worked a full week, they were not regarded as full-time workers, eligible for benefits. Hardly any of the union members thought of the union as a place to turn for redress of their grievances, though, of course, they enjoyed greater security and more protection than the nonunion people.

I suppose one could make a case for the employer changing a patient's benefits or insurance on the grounds of increased cost or risk, a weak case, but a case. A study done at the Mayo Clinic in 1977 makes such a case. Surveying patients and insurers to determine possible cancer-related discrimination, it found that 208 of 940 patient respondents claimed instances of discrimination, almost all (90 percent) of which concerned insurance, especially applications for new or additional coverage. The study concludes that the use of increased premiums and exclusions of coverage were "reasonable," the industry considers them sound practices. The cancellation of insurance and refusals of application were judged "less reasonable acts."

However, it is hard to excuse another kind of discrimination. This is the hostility, grounded in ignorance and fear, shown the returned cancer patient: mimicry, shunning, caustic or sarcastic comments, teasing. The hanger-in experiences them all to some degree, the blue collar workers more than the white collar, and the young people going back to school much more than their peers going back to work. Sometimes it was subtle, "The school counselor I got sent to by the teacher didn't want to *talk* to me; he wanted to *pray* with me," said a junior high school student. Often it was not. "At school," said the mother of a seventeen-year-old, "he was treated like a freak! I wouldn't have the courage or strength to endure what he did."

"I thought things were different when I returned to work," explained one blue collar woman. "The people there seemed less friendly and tried to avoid me. Maybe they thought I was 'catchy.' I didn't really want to go back. Some of them visited me at the hospital, but I already knew about the feelings people have about cancer. It upsets a lot of people."

The interviewers felt that especially the unskilled and semi-

144

skilled workers, may have projected onto the work place their own long-established views that people with this dread disease were to be abhorred. This enhanced their own shame and intensified their hostility to others.

Be that as it may, many could not separate their distress about treatment by coworkers from their feelings about other matters. They worried about finances and insurance benefits for themselves and their survivors, the blue collar workers more than the white collar ones with more resources. They feared reduced or cancelled group health insurance if they changed jobs, or if their illness—or any other illness or incapacity—would develop.

How would their families meet such costs? How would their surviving dependents be protected with life insurance not available in the work place? How would their families do when the wife or husband could no longer cling to the job and they were dependent on one income?

Hostility at work, whether real or imagined, contributed to the workers' emotional distress. This distress was heightened if the patient had failed to seek and use medical advice as soon as symptoms appeared. This was particularly true of breast cancer patients. One reported she was aware of new lumps but had not been able to see the doctor: she was "needed" on the job. Deeply anxious, especially since her mother had died two years before, she said she feared to be absent: If she lost this job, where would she get another? Would she be able to work?

If their doctors had been unaware of the seriousness of their symptoms, as was true of 10 percent of the white collar patients, most of them with head-neck or colo-rectal cancer, the patients' anger almost always turned on the doctor, rather than themselves. Many wanted mental health counseling; many feared that they might loose coverage for it. Their distress about this and other matters overflowed and was expressed in the work place, especially when they became aware of symptoms; when they decided to consult the doctor; when the decision to carry out the medical recommendation was made; when cancer was confirmed; upon return to the job; and sometimes, when a work

145

crisis occurred. As a blue collar employer put it, "She drove everyone crazy with her harping on how she felt and what she was afraid would have to be done." He refused to rehire her.

The kind of medical care these hanging-in patients received was crucial. The young people especially wanted information directly from their doctors but often got it instead through their parents. The doctor's perception of the work place and the worker's realistic position there was important, "The doctor sent in a statement that 'blew it'—not in what he *wrote* but how it was interpreted that (this Hodgkin's disease patient) was a 'high risk'."

An interesting pattern could be seen among the blue collar workers: combinations of low income, delay in seeking medical care, particularly poor experiences with the medical care obtained (one doctor, for example, delayed giving treatment as long as four years), and physically demanding occupations.

At the other end of the scale were patients who made quick recoveries, worked many hours of overtime in physically strenuous jobs, or concurrently carried two or even three additional jobs. Usually they were in less menial jobs, had gotten early medical care of unquestionable quality, had comfortable incomes, and their personalities were such that they could plan realistically.

From all this you can see why employees, fearing jeopardy of seniority, insurance benefits, and pension rights and harrassed both medically and on the job, feel frightened of the future. Many in the studies went job hunting, nearly half of the blue collar workers, for example. There was evidence that almost 70 percent of them would have liked to look for another job if they weren't so worried about gatekeepers, like personnel officers, or examining physicians, excluding them or preventing them from gaining equal benefits in a new position.

To rectify these fears and make the work place a safer place for recovered patients, Dr. Frances Feldman recommends many improvements. She would like, for example, to see medical

146

counseling services established, especially for young workers in need of information and its interpretation. She would like to see vocational counseling to help workers deal realistically with alternative jobs and occupations, understand and deal with work-place problems, and prepare for applications. She would like to see more personal and mental health counseling and a great deal more medical and public education to acquaint people with the special needs and situations of hanging-in patients. She would like to see bridges built between employers and service providers, like counselors.

I say amen to all of this. I would work particularly hard with the doctors, a target group in this complicated picture, relatively easy to reach, and often anxious to be more helpful. Usually they vaguely tell patients, "Do what you feel like doing," which leaves everyone confused as to whether someone can work and, if so, exactly what the limitations are.

Back to the old doctor-communications problem, which I have belabored before. It is true that as Lawrence D. Burke, Rehabilitation Director at the National Cancer Institute, puts it, "The work place is therapeutic for us. My wife does not love me because I'm handsome or rich, but because I work." In Burke's experience, many employers in need of workers realize this but are unsure from equivocal medical reports just what to expect of hanging-in patients.

In the same way, the patients themselves are confused, so cannot take complete responsibility for their actions. Until they do, they cannot take legal action to redress their grievances. The rights of cancer patients in certain work situations are protected by the Rehabilitation Act of 1973, though few of them know about it (including me, until I did the research for this book).

This federal law protects a handicapped patient who has "any impairment which substantially limits one or more of a person's major life activities," and a hanging-in cancer patient is such a person. Section 503 of the act requires major federal contractors and subcontractors to prepare and maintain affirmative action programs for the handicapped, to recruit, hire, and promote qualified handicapped workers. Under this section, a patient with cancer of the larynx, for instance, might be entitled to speech therapy, counseling, "socialization"—with Lost Chord Clubs and others, and recreation services. The broader Section 504 prohibits discrimination against the handicapped person by certain employers receiving federal assistance.

Complaints against those defined in both sections of the act can be filed (for 503, with the U.S. Department of Labor's Office of Federal Contract Compliance Practices; for 504, with the Department of Human Resources' Office of Civil Rights). But, as I say, not many people know about this. The generally optimistic study done at the Mayo Clinic mentioned before found only a minority of cancer patients surveyed (15 percent) are aware of their eligibility for vocational rehabilitation services.

Two vignettes:
• A decade ago, I sat in on a training program for "environmental technicians" (garbage men) to gather material for an article. Later, my teacher-friend Helen Mitchell and I put on green Department of Sanitation uniforms and went out on the garbage trucks, throwing trash with her pupils.

It was back-breaking, dirty labor, out there in the trash-filled alleys often with mangy dogs barking at our heels, but it was work, it was life. Remembering Memphis, one man told me, "Martin Luther King died for us." In the same sense, as we see in the next chapter, every hanging-in patient dies for every other and wants to leave a record to take pride in.

• A month after his surgery, wrote Hubert Humphrey, he went back to work, for he felt there is nothing worse than for someone with something like cancer to have nothing to do.

People told him he should cut down on his schedule, but he knew it was important to be involved with people and activities. He enjoyed being a senator. When he was at committee meetings, handling major issues, talking away, he felt part of the life of this country. He felt alive.

To feel alive. To work. That is what all of us want and need.

CHAPTER 10

THE BIG PICTURE: SEARCH FOR MEANING

To feel, to be alive. When Ivan Ilych, the hero of Tolstoi's great short story, lay dying, he listened to the voice of his own soul, to the current of thoughts rising within him.

"What do you want?" this voice asked. "What do you want?"

"What do I want? To live and not to suffer."

"To live? How?" asked his inner voice.

"Why, to live as I used to, well and pleasantly."

"As you lived before, well and pleasantly?"

I had read and reread *The Death of Ivan Ilych* many times. In fact, I had used the "to live and not to suffer" phrase repeatedly during my Department of Health, Education and Welfare speech writing days, to capsule what patients want out of our health care system.

Until my cancer experience, I never completely understood how Ivan, and Leo Tolstoi, felt as he lay on his couch, reviewing his life and seeking its meaning. Until then, like Ivan, I knew that "Caius is a man, men are mortal, therefore Caius is mortal." Like Ivan, I knew that syllogism was correct as applied to the abstract Caius, "but certainly not as applied to himself" (myself).

Now, like other patients in my position, I could no longer dismiss my own mortality. One day, perhaps sooner than later, I might not be alive. I could hope, I did hope, but my end would actually come. I had to ask myself: "What did it mean to die? To live? Was I making best use of what time I had left? As Susan Sontag explains her own sense of urgency when she developed cancer, "Death becomes quite real to you, and you never return to that more innocent relation to life you had before. It really makes having priorities and trying to follow them very real to you."

Early on in my illness, I remember telling my friend Nancy Harrison that I was spending perhaps too much time mulling over my situation. She had been hanging in much longer than I with breast cancer, and she told me that at the beginning she too often just sat on the couch weaving the psychic threads together, trying to figure it all out. Her husband, Gil, (then editor of *The New Republic*) had sometimes felt "enough's enough," but for her all the figuring out hours were not time wasted. When her illness recurred she became more and more active in St. Alban's Church, giving to her faith and gaining from it, cramming more and more into each day: one more church seminar, one more lecture, one more inner-city school project. Many felt that this engaging woman, outstanding as she had been as a philanthropist and education leader, and successful as she had been as a wife and mother, was never so serene and fulfilled as in the last years of her life.

Not all hanging-in patients can treat their experience as a challenge and use it to grow and find personal meaning. But if they can do so, it makes a difference. California Chief Justice Rose Elizabeth Bird has reported that after her first bout with cancer, she had denied the possibility of recurrence and submerged herself in her work. Its recurrence was an illuminating experience, "In a peculiar way," she told a Los Angeles medical forum "death can teach you what life is all about. It is a painful lesson and a difficult journey, but I am personally grateful that I was made to travel this path at a relatively early age."

Her gratitude, Justice Bird explained, stemmed from the

150

increased time she had to learn much about herself, much about how precious life and people are to her, and to modify her behavior in various ways, so that she could, for example, eat in a more healthy way or try to deal more effectively with the stresses in her life. In short, she had time to do what the Bishop in Margaret Craven's lyrical novel, *I Heard the Owl Call My Name*, told his young minister-protegé was the great benefit of living in the remote seacoast village of Kingcome, B.C., among the Kwakiutl Indians, where only the fundamentals count: to learn enough of the meaning of life to be ready to die.

I too am thankful I have had hanging-in time—not enough, perhaps, but more, I suspect, than my doctors expected. At the begining, I, like Rose Bird, took the workaholic road. Whenever I found myself sitting and stewing, my anxiety about my future, or lack of it, increasing, I simply accepted another writing assignment or went looking for a consultant job. My first recurrence did not force a radical change; that seldom happens. It did cause me to try, at least, to examine my inchoate views of God and man, to try to reach some firmer conviction about the core of our existence.

In chapter 5, I reported about the way I wept at Sloan-Kettering, mourning the black hole, the nothingness, of my mortality as I talked to Sister Rosemary. Back home, I floundered in my quest for answers to eternal riddles. It seemed to me that the religious people were the lucky ones. I envied their strong, clear faith, their ready access to language and symbols on which they could lean.

When she was told she had a good year to live, perhaps five or six more, with treatment, Marvella Bayh could ask with the old hymn, "Where could I go, but to the Lord?" She turned to her neighbor, a born-again Christian, for help in learning how to believe, to plug into God's healing love, to trust, to hope for a miracle, and to give her strength to further His work, through her own. My hospital roommate, Aunt Jemima kerchief on her head and Medicaid card in her pocketbook, had far fewer earthly resources than I. But she had Jesus at her side, and she

151

knew he was in there, pitching for her. My friend Nancy could forcefully challenge the young minister who was teaching the St. Alban's "Death" seminar she had organized when he dared to suggest that death might indeed be the end for us, and that it was a mark of unselfish maturity to recognize and accept this. So strong was the opposition of those of our classmates who believed in some sort of resurrection, who were sure that an organized universe could not countenance lost souls, that he was made to recant at the next session.

But I was left with him, uncertain and in doubt. I would have preferred to feel, like many men and women I know, that I would be rewarded in the next life if I endured suffering courageously, if I took up my cross with faith. Instead, I found myself a casualty of a rational and scientific modern age, wondering if there were any meaning to my pain. Turning to Judaism, my own religion, I found myself comfortable with the most skeptical of Old Testament authors, Ecclesiastes, who applied his heart to know wisdom and concluded, "Whatsoever thy hand findeth to do, do it with all thy might; for there is no work, no device, nor knowledge, nor wisdom, in Sheol [the grave], whither thou goest."

Ecclesiastes understood the search for meaning, but warns off people like me who search too hard: "He hath made everything beautiful in its time," he tells us, "also he hath set eternity in their heart, yet so that man cannot find out the work that God hath done, from the beginning even to the end." That man cannot find out, the work that God hath done. Perhaps this is so.

Bernard Mehlman, then Rabbi of the little teaching congregation to which we belong in Washington, Temple Micah, called on me in the fall of 1977. We talked, I wept, and he recommended to me "The Heart Determines," Martin Buber's interpretation of Psalm 73. Later, he sent me *Good and Evil*, the Buber book in which this essay appears. I read and reread it, finding in it each time a reaffirmation of a suspicion: that the Old Testament, which exhorts us in such a magnificent way to choose life—the blessing rather than the curse—and would have us live it justly, mercifully, and humbly, offers us faint comfort in death.

152

For the essay, which seems to me to reflect the thinking more of Buber, the modern philosopher, than the Biblical Psalmist, explains that over against the realm of nothing, Sheol, there is God. The Psalmist does not aspire to enter heaven after death; there is nothing here about this ("And so far as I see," adds Buber, "there is nothing in the Old Testament about this."). But he knows he will soon be wholly with Him who "has taken" him. He does not mean by this what we are accustomed to call personal immortality. His heart, the inmost organ of his soul, will vanish with his flesh when he vanishes in death. Only the true part and true fate of this person, the "rock" of his heart, God, is eternal. Into this eternity he who is pure in heart moves in death. This eternity is something absolutely different from any familiar mortal kind of time.

I got the same message, in somewhat simpler, more traditional form, a few years after Rabbi Mehlman introduced me to the Buber essay. My old friend and neighbor Hadassah, or "Handy," Davis dropped by during a visit to Washington. As we sat in the garden, talking, I told her about my search and my feeling that the Old Testament offered less to the person facing death than the New, with its personification of God, its cross, and its resurrection. She said she would ask her father, Rabbi Louis Finkelstein, to write to me. I was delighted. I would be enlightened by one of the most renowned Jewish scholars, the distinguished Rabbi who had headed the Jewish Theological Seminary of America.

Handy kept her word. Her father's letter arrived at the end of 1979. Louis Finkelstein wrote that all Jewish authorities who were and are in the tradition have held that immortality of the soul is a basic dogma and that our stay here on earth is merely a prelude to a blessed and happy life. The reason that the biblical prophets avoided speaking of human mortality and resurrection of the dead is that, like most primitive peoples, the surrounding peoples of their time worshipped the dead. Since this was considered idolatry, they were hesitant to refer to the dead as still being alive. After the exile, this danger became remote, and thus leaders felt free to speak of human immortality.

153

Both in his letter to me and in a copy of one he enclosed to his granddaughter, Rabbi Finkelstein explained that from the Jews the doctrine of immortality was taken over by the Christian and Moslem philosophers to become the basic doctrine of all Western religion, as well as by philosophers like Socrates and Plato, and in modern times, William James and A. N. Whitehead. Obviously, he argued, there is no way of demonstrating such a doctrine in the scientific laboratory, but it seemed difficult for him to understand how a belief that is so widespread and makes so much sense out of the riddle of human existence, can be rejected. Death could not be very far off for him, but it was nothing to be worried about because it would be like going from one room to another, only that in that second room, there are no troubles, no pains, no sickness, only joy and the opportunity to study. I heard the same thing at Arkansas Congressman Brooks Hays' funeral last year from a prominent Baptist minister: Brooks, the famed hero of Little Rock, had retired upstairs to sleep; we would be joining him later.

Rabbi Finkelstein concluded that he had known many skeptics, but most had their belief hidden away somewhere in the back of their minds. Justice Felix Frankfurter, for instance, earnestly asked that the Kaddish be said when he died, and it was done. Well, I, too, want the Kaddish, the great mourner's prayer, which does not mention death, said when I die; I want to be part of the continuity of the generations. I, too, have some sort of belief hidden away at the back of my mind. But it seemed to me that the Rabbi was asking me to accept on faith that my soul would be unaffected by my death, simply because so many people smarter than I had done so. He didn't mention that other people smarter than I had not done so.

As I struggled to attain Sontag's "less innocent relationship to life," reading and taking another "Death" course, I found practical comfort in the work of a physician-poet whose feet, at least, are planted firmly in the scientific laboratory, Lewis Thomas. In The Medussa and the Snail, Dr. Thomas explains that he used to wince at the sight of a dying field mouse in the jaws of an amiable household cat. Now he wonders if his dying is necessarily different from the overnight passing of a backyard elm, struck down by lightning, which has no pain receptors. At the instant of the mouse's being trapped and penetrated by teeth, peptide hormones are released by cells in the hypothalamus and pituitary gland; instantly these "endorphins" are attached to the surfaces of the other cells responsible for pain perceptions; the hormones have the pharmacological properties of opium; there is no pain. So when it's end game, pain, which is useful for avoidance when there's still time to get away, is likely to be turned off, precisely and quickly, and the animal slides into death; if he could shrug, he would shrug. If Dr. Thomas were to design an ecosystem in which creatures had to live off each other and dying were an indispensable part of living, he could think of no better way to manage.

Nor can I. This awe at the miraculous workings of the Grand Design represents the limits of my understanding at this time. I cannot let go of it. As the author John Updike said recently, "I've never let it go, because when the faith goes, I never could see any other consolation." I don't belittle those who can take it a step, even a leap, further toward a less abstract faith. On the contrary, I envy them.

Asked if I was afraid of dying on the PBS television show, "A Different Kind of Life," I answered truthfully that though I might pretend not to be, as our macho culture seems to demand, I was as afraid as everyone else. But billions of people have lived in this world, and billions have died; I could see no reason why I might be different from them, under whatever rules there are.

At the same conference where I met Harry, the blind jogger, whom we encountered in chapter 5, I came across a notion that helped enormously in my personal search for meaning. It was posited by California's Charles A. Garfield, a psychologist working with seriously ill patients. To learn about life in the extremity of life-threatening illness, he said, he had turned to the literature of the Holocaust. Referring to Terrence Des Pres' remarkable book, *The Survivor: An Anatomy of Life in the*

Death Camps, he drew several important analogies between the two lives. In both, for instance, the extreme situation is not an event, nor a crisis with a beginning, middle, or end, but simply a state of existence without the encouragement of visible progress or positive end in sight, and always with the knowledge that death may win.

This is true. Still, the idea of comparing my situation with that of a Holocaust victim seemed a bit pretentious, at first. I have not, after all, been beaten with whips, worn ragged clothing torn by dogs, breathed air so foul from excremental assault that no bird flew overhead. My hanging-in experiences seemed trivial contrasted to these humiliating horrors.

I walked around the corner to our congenial neighborhood Francis Scott Key Bookstore and placed an order for the Des Pres book. While I waited for it to arrive, I reread Victor E. Frankl's compelling account of his own concentration camp experiences, in *Man's Search for Meaning.*

When it came, *The Survivor,* which compiles actual testimony of survivors of Russian as well as Nazi death camps, fiercely and movingly underlined what I had acknowledged rereading Frankl through my newly found survivors' glasses. Indeed, there were many significant parallels between the hanging-in and the camp experiences, not so much in the terrible damage done to the human body in both worlds—nothing could equal the naked vilification of the Holocaust—as in the intensification of the inner life of those trapped there and the clues this provided to the art of survival.

In the first place, and this blew my mind when I read it, there was in the death camps, as Elie Wiesel put it, "a veritable passion to testify." The Holocaust produced an endless scream, which in time was heard in the voices of an unusual number of literate witnesses. Men and women knew they had to survive to leave a trace, to tell people how they lived and died; they had to survive to make the deathly silence speak, to erect a memorial to millions of bodies burned in the gas chambers. At Treblenka, they prepared to destroy the camp so as to allow at least one man or woman to live to tell the tale; forty survived. Two men,

156

Michael Berg and Alexander Donat accidently switched places in a death brigade; Berg wrote *The Holocaust Kingdom* in Donat's name.

The analogy to the hanging-in experience struck me forcibly. "Death is compounded by oblivion," Des Pres explains, "and the foundation of humanness—faith in continuity—is endangered." Why else do so many of us hanging-in patients tell our stories through articles, books, and TV shows? In cancer support groups, clinic waiting rooms, hospital corridors, over the telephone after I had published a newspaper piece, I have met men and women who write, or want to write about their experiences. Unlike the death camp survivors, they cannot hope by so doing to prevent a future repetition of all their sufferings; they cannot cry "Never Again!" But like those other survivors, they can show that they were *there* and that what happened to them mattered. They can show their compassion for those who did not make it and their loyalty. They can try to help others by leaving them hints as to how to survive.

For both, lives lived in extremity are collective acts. In the camps, men and women were reduced to a single mass of bone-thin festering bodies with shaved heads, clad in filthy rags. They depended on each other for survival, propping up comrades when they lagged, exhausted and barefooted in the snow, hiding each other from brutal guards, smuggling food to satisfy each other's hunger. In hanging-in places too, be they a "Magic Mountain" sanatorium, or Sloan-Kettering, patients with bald heads and often mutilated bodies share a social identity. They support each other, exchanging information rather than food.

Of all their advantages, none is more crucial than the fact that their caretakers want to help, rather than hurt them. The SS guards took pleasure in telling Dachau inmates that they had no chance of coming out alive, and after the war the world would not believe what had happened. Our doctors, nurses, and counselors take pleasure, some with more success than others, in encouraging us to hope and to survive.

Victor Frankl tells how a wise senior block warden asked him

157

to address his fellow prisoners at the end of a bad day in the camps. A semistarved prisoner had broken into a store to steal a few pounds of potatoes. Other prisoners had recognized the culprit, and the authorities ordered that the guilty man be given up, "Naturally, the 2,500 men preferred to starve."

Though he was cold and hungry, psychiatrist Frankl recognized an opportunity to encourage his comrades, lying about him, wan and exhausted on the earthen hut floor. Even in the sixth winter of the Second World War, he pointed out, their situation was not the most terrible they could imagine. After all, their bones were intact, they were still alive. They had reason to hope that health, family, fortune, happiness, professional careers would be restored.

No man, Frankl continued, knew what the future would bring. Though there was still no typhus in the camp, he estimated his own chances of surviving at about one in twenty. Still, he had no intention of losing hope, of giving up. Something might open up, the luck of attachment, for example, to a special group with good working conditions.

Turning to the past, the psychiatrist argued that no power on earth could take away what they had experienced, all they had suffered; even their seemingly hopeless struggle had dignity and meaning. He quoted Nietzche: "That which does not kill me makes me stronger."

Those with any religious faith could understand the man who bargained with God that his suffering should save the person he loved. Like other men and women, he did not want to die for nothing. In difficult times, someone looks down on each of us, a God, a friend, a wife. That someone will be disappointed if we do not know how to die, suffering, not miserably, but proudly.

They were still alive, their bones intact. No intention of losing hope, something might open up. To die suffering proudly. Even in the most abnormal of lives in extremity, the way in which you deal with fate, the attitude with which you take up the cross, gives deeper meaning to the days you have. Those who can step toward this deeper meaning and perform the acts of life accordingly often have the best chance for survival. This is as true in the hanging in as in the death camp experience.

Entering either of these unreal, provisional existences from which there is no set release date, human beings can be shocked to the point of collapse. Terrorized, mourning, lacking information about what to do or how to act, you can lose your desire to fight for life with all your being. Lost in the nightmare of the Holocaust, time ran out on the *Muselmänner* (Moslems) as the "walking dead" were called. They died before they were able to shake off their terrorized shock, wake to their predicament, and fight it. Lost in the perceived nightmare of hanging-in treatment, the patient can also give up and die quite soon.

Those who survive can build a wall of apathy around themselves, denying that what is all about them is really happening. This has its own dangers: Though apathy may keep despair at a distance, it may result in disregard for the environment, so that neither prisoner nor patient strives to adapt to it. Fortunately, in both worlds many emerge from apathy to fight as best they can, refusing to see their "victimization" as total.

They renew this stubborn will each morning, not through what Terrence Des Pres calls, "some secret fortitude of the heart," but through the physical act of getting up, either from a few hours of death camp sleep, or from a troubled sick bed. The pain might be great, the misery deep, but the commitment to another day must be made. An Auschwitz survivor reports the sores on his feet opened as he climbed down and put on his shoes each morning; he knew a new day had begun. Similarly, I have often felt, putting my luckier feet into my slippers after a bad night, recommitted to another stretch of existence. Also, I have on occasion asked like Solzhenitsyn's Kostoglotov entering the cancer ward for treatment that would deprive him of his virility, "Isn't that an exorbitant price? Should I pay it?"

Extremity deepens relationships, intensifies social bonding. Survivors depend more on others; in fact, survival is, as we have noted, a collective act. No one survives without help; many find great joy in service to others. The camp inmates were

159

necessarily dependent on each other, for a little extra food, protection from the guards, advice as to how to find a clerking job, even for physical guidance when struck by night blindness (a frequent illness among vitamin-starved prisoners in northern camps).

From each other they asked not pity, nor sentimentality, but support and camaraderie. One of their delights was giving each other gifts—a potato, a leaf, a piece of string. The more fortunate hanging-in patient can turn for help to a wealth of sources: family, friends, caretakers, as well as fellows in support groups. We, too, ask less for pity, or sympathy, than for proof of friendship and caring. An outpouring of love and affection from her multitude of friends was a source of deep satisfaction to Diana Michaelis in the final days of her hanging in. Even as this woman with a genuine gift for friendship lay almost comatose, she smiled at each visitor and tried to discuss politics or world affairs with them. Many among us find deep satisfaction in trying to help others: Marvella Bayh, on the speaking circuit during the last year of her life, for example, or Terese Lasser, who founded the national volunteer visiting organization, Reach to Recovery, after her mastectomy experience.

But a contradiction exists. Though we survive by helping one another, both death camp prisoners and hanging-in patients know it is every man, every woman, for himself. The prisoners learned how to work for, or even in, camp administration, how to curry small favors from the authorities, realistically and without illusion. A strong sense of self-hood, of personhood helped. Esther Milgrom, my friend Toby Levin's mother, tells how she escaped from a long line of naked prisoners bound for the gas chambers at Auschwitz. She sighted a pile of clothes near a barracks and knew that she, a self-respecting human being, *should be wearing them;* once clothed, she became lost in a crowd of laborers. Later, she remembers keeping the little floor space that was hers spotless, a dignified shiny-clean.

Less dramatically, we hanging-in patients learn how to deal with doctors and other caretakers who influence our lives. We learn firmly to distance ourselves from people whom we upset,

160

or who upset us. We learn to undertake only those tasks we can do realistically and to try to keep ourselves attractively groomed (you can always tell those sad "shades," as Diana called them, in the clinics, who have given up). If we don't watch out for ourselves, who will?

Life goes on, even at its extreme limits. It rises up, sinks down, in a definite rhythm of decline and renewal. Survivors awake and reawake, fall low and begin to die, return to life, as much in long-time illness as in the death camps. All must run risks that bring them closer to death to stay alive. A prisoner decided that he would not be afraid of camp labor, but would risk slowly, tenaciously dragging himself through the twelve-hour day. Esther Milgrom had the guts to help more fearful prisoners risk approaching the guards for a little extra food or clothing. I, like many other patients, decide to risk yet another difficult operation, or undergo chemotherapy to gain more quality time.

Those who have a sense of humor have a definite advantage. Recognizing that humor offers the ability to rise above a situation, if only briefly, and thus is one of the soul's weapons in the fight for self-preservation, Victor Frankl suggested to a surgeon friend that they tell each other an amusing story every day. Hubert Humphrey stalked the Sloan-Kettering corridors in his bathrobe, joshing and encouraging fellow patients, telling jokes.

Those who can find a kind of negative happiness in their situation have an advantage, too. They can say, with Dr. Frankl, that things are not as terrible as one would imagine, they could be worse. They can find joy in a lovely tree branch, or intricate flower, or rainbow sunset. They can delight in working rhythmically and skillfully with a squad to build a wall in the freezing cold, or writing well, even in a sickbed. They can believe something—deliverance from the Holocaust, a cure for cancer—will turn up. In fact, the function of intelligence in extremity seems not so much to judge your chances, which may be almost zero (those cancer statistics again), as to make the most of the opportunity of getting through each day.

161

Some succeed in helping others unselfishly, others simply develop their talent for life, their ability to rely on the power of life itself. But both in the death camp and the hanging-in clinic, survivors stand firm, acknowledging the centrality of death, yet choosing life; taking their stand right on the line, staying there, hanging in, even when their will to go on may seem illogical. In this way the ordeal of the survivor becomes an experience of growth and self-realization.

SELECTED BIBLIOGRAPHY

(Used as sources for this book)

Ahmed, Paul, ed. *Living and Dying with Cancer.* New York: Elsevier, 1981.

Alsop, Stewart. *Stay of Execution.* New York: Harper and Row, 1973.

Bayh, Marvella with Kotz, Mary Lynn. *Marvella.* New York: Harcourt Brace Jovanovich, 1979.

Beattie, Edward J. with Cowan, Stuart D. *Toward the Conquest of Cancer.* New York: Crown Publishers, Inc., 1980.

Buber, Martin. *Good and Evil.* New York: Scribners, 1952.

Cantor, Robert Cherin. *And a Time To Live.* New York: Harper and Row, 1978.

Cassell, Eric L. *The Healer's Art.* New York and Philadelphia: J. B. Lippincott, Co., 1979.

Cassileth, Barrie R. *The Cancer Patient.* Philadelphia: Lea and Febiger, 1979.

Chemotherapy and You—A Guide to Self-Help During Treatment. Bethesda, MD: National Cancer Institute (NIH Publication No. 81-1136), 1980.

Coelho, George V.; Hamburg, David A.; and Adams, John E., eds. *Coping and Adaptation.* New York: Basic Books, 1974.

Coping With Cancer: A Resource for the Health Professional. Bethesda, MD: National Cancer Institute, 1980.

Craven, Margaret. *I Heard the Owl Call My Name.* New York: Doubleday, 1973.

Crile, George, Jr. *What Women Should Know About The Breast Cancer Controversy.* New York: Pocket Books, 1974.

Cullen, Joseph W.; Fox, Bernard H.; and Isom, Ruby N. *Cancer, The Behavioral Dimensions.* New York: Raven Press, 1976.

Des Pres, Terrence. *The Survivor: An Anatomy of Life in the Death Camps.* New York: Oxford University Press, 1976.

Feldman, Frances Lomas. *Work and Cancer Health Histories— A Study of the Experiences of Recovered Patients.* San Francisco: California Division, American Cancer Society, 1976.

_____. *Work and Cancer Health Histories—A Study of the Experiences of Blue Collar Workers.* San Francisco: California Division, American Cancer Society, 1978.

_____. *Work and Cancer Health Histories—Work Expectations and Experiences of Youth (Ages 13-23) with Cancer Histories.* Oakland: California Division, American Cancer Society, 1980.

Frank, Jerome. *Persuasion and Healing.* Baltimore: The Johns Hopkins University Press, 1961.

Frankl, Victor E. *Man's Search For Meaning.* New York: Pocket Books, 1963.

Garfield, Charles A. *Stress and Survival.* St. Louis: The C.V. Mosby Co., 1979.

Hutschnecker, Arnold. *Hope.* New York: G.P. Putnam, 1981.

Israël, Lucien. *Conquering Cancer.* New York: Random House, 1978.

Johnson, Thomas J. (selector). *Emily Dickinson's Poems.* Boston: Little Brown and Co., 1961.

Kübler-Ross, Elisabeth. *On Death and Dying.* New York: Macmillan Publishing Co., 1969.

Kushner, Rose. *Why Me? Newly Rewritten for the Eighties.* New York, The Saunders Press, 1982.

Lange, Arthur J., and Jakubowski, Patricia. *Responsible Assertive Behavior.* Champaign, IL: Research Press, 1976.

LeShan, Lawrence. *You Can Fight For Your Life.* New York: M. Evans and Co., 1977.

Listen to the Children! New York: Cancer Care and the National Cancer Foundation, 1977.

Mayo Clinic Rehabilitation Program. *A Study of Discrimination Toward Cancer Patients by Insurers, Employers and Vocational Rehabilitation Agencies.* Rochester, MN: The Vocational Insurance Committee, Mayo Clinic Rehabilitation Program, October, 1977.

Morra, Marion, and Potts, Eve. *Choices: Realistic Alternatives in Cancer Treatment.* New York: Avon Books, 1980.

Power, Paul W., and Dell Orto, Arthur E., eds. *Role of the Family in the Rehabilitation of the Physically Disabled.* Baltimore: University Park Press, 1980.

Proceedings of the American Cancer Society's National Conference on Human Values and Cancer. Atlanta, June 22–24, 1972.

Proceedings of the American Cancer Society's Second National Conference on Human Values and Cancer. Chicago, September 7–9, 1977.

Proceedings of the American Cancer Society's Third National Conference on Human Values and Cancer. Washington, D.C., April 23–25, 1981.

Radiation Therapy and You—A Guide to Self-Help During Treatment. Bethesda, MD: National Cancer Institute (NHI Publication No. 80-2227), 1980.

Rosenbaum, Ernest H., and Isadora R. *A Comprehensive Guide for Cancer Patients and Their Families.* Palo Alto: Bull Publishing Co., 1980.

Select Committee on Aging. *Frontiers in Cancer Research for the Elderly,* (96th Cong., 1st Sess.) Washington, D.C.: U.S. Government Printing Office (Serial No. 96-61), 1979.

Select Committee on Aging. *Cancer Insurance: Exploiting Fear for Profit,* (96th Cong., 2nd Sess.) Washington, D.C.: U.S.

Government Printing Office (Comm. Pub. No. 96-202), 1980.

Simonton, O. Carl; Simonton, Stephanie Matthews; and Creighton, James. *Getting Well Again.* Los Angeles: J.P. Tarcher, Inc., 1978.

Sontag, Susan. *Illness as Metaphor.* New York: Random House, 1978.

Strain, James J., and Grossman, Stanley, *Psychological Care of the Medically Ill: A Primer in Liaison Psychiatry.* New York: Appleton-Century-Crofts, 1975.

Taking Time: Support for People with Cancer and the People Who Care About Them. Bethesda, MD: National Cancer Institute, 1980.

Terkel, Studs. *Working.* New York: Pantheon, 1974.

The Psychological Impact of Cancer. New York: American Cancer Society, Professional Education Publication, 1954.

There is a Rainbow Behind Every Cloud. Tiburon, CA: Center for Attitudinal Healing, 1978.

Thomas, Lewis. *The Lives of a Cell.* New York: The Viking Press, 1974.

_____. *The Medusa and the Snail.* New York: The Viking Press, 1979.

Tolstoi, Leo. *The Death of Ivan Ilych.* London: Oxford University Press, 1935; Chicago: The Great Books Foundation, 1955.

Van Skoy-Mosher, Michael, ed. *Controversies in Cancer Treatment.* Boston: G. K. Hall Co., 1981.

Walter, Carol with Miller, Leonore. *A Total Program of Post Mastectomy Exercises.* New York: The Bobbs-Merrill Co., 1981.

Weaver, Peter. *Strategies for the Second Half of Life.* New York: New American Library (Signet), 1981.

Weisman, Avery D. *Coping with Cancer.* New York: McGraw-Hill Book Co., 1979.

INDEX

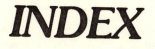

168

362.1
Sp46h

Spingarn.
Ha~~nging~~ in there.

362.1
Sp46h

Spingarn.
Hanging in there.

DATE	ISSUED TO	
MAY 1 8 1983	*Cheryl Kudena*	*milligan #13*
6-24-83	*~~Jason Stevenson~~*	
	Mildred Giesler	
1-10-84	*Mildred Reinke*	*icc*
FEB 23 1984	*FEB 2*~~~~	